Guided Self-Rehabilitation
Contract in Spastic Paresis

Jean-Michel Gracies

Guided Self-Rehabilitation Contract in Spastic Paresis

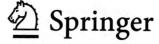

Jean-Michel Gracies
Paris, France

ISBN 978-3-319-29107-9   ISBN 978-3-319-29108-6   (eBook)
https://doi.org/10.1007/978-3-319-29108-6

Responsible Editor: Corinna Parravicini
This Springer imprint is published by the registered company Springer Nature
Switzerland AG
The registered company address is: Gewerbestrasse 11, 6330 Cham, Switzerland

Contents

Author biography   IX

Foreword   XII

Understanding spastic paresis...   XII

Introduction   XVI

Neuroloco   XVII

PART ONE: LOWER LIMB ANATOMICAL REVIEW   1

HIP

1   Gluteus maximus – Passive stretch   5

2   Gluteus maximus – Active hip flexion, knee flexed   7

3   Hamstrings – Passive stretch   9

4   Hamstrings – Active hip flexion, knee extended   11

5   Hip flexor-adductors – Passive stretch   13

6   Hip extensor-adductors – Passive stretch   15

7   Hip adductors – Active hip abduction   17

8   Hip internal rotators – Passive stretch   19

9   Hip internal rotators – Active hip external rotation   21

KNEE

10   Rectus femoris – Passive stretch   23

11   Rectus femoris – Active knee flexion, hip extended   25

12   Vastus muscles – Passive stretch   27

13   Vastus muscles – Active knee flexion, hip flexed   29

ANKLE

14 **Soleus – Passive stretch**   31

15 **Soleus – Active ankle dorsiflexion, seated**   33

16 **Gastrocnemius** (medial and lateral) **– Passive stretch**   35

17 **Gastrocnemius – Active ankle dorsiflexion, standing**   37

LOWER LIMB FUNCTIONAL EXERCISES

18 **Sit-to-stand**   39

19 **Long stride walking**   41

20 **Fast walking**   43

PART TWO: UPPER LIMB ANATOMICAL REVIEW

SHOULDER

21 **Pectoralis major – Passive stretch**   51

22 **Pectoralis major – Active shoulder abduction**   53

23 **Latissimus dorsi and long head of triceps – Passive stretch**   55

24 **Latissimus dorsi – Active shoulder flexion, elbow extended**   57

25 **Long head of triceps – Active shoulder flexion, elbow flexed**   59

26 **Sub-scapularis – Passive stretch**   61

27 **Sub-scapularis – Active shoulder external rotation**   63

ELBOW

28 **Elbow flexors – Passive stretch**   65

29 **Elbow flexors – Active elbow extension**   67

30 Pronator quadratus – Passive stretch   **69**

31 Pronator quadratus – Active supination, elbow flexed   **71**

32 Pronator teres – Passive stretch   **73**

33 Pronator teres – Active supination, elbow extended   **75**

WRIST

34 Wrist flexors – Passive stretch   **77**

35 Wrist flexors – Active wrist extension   **79**

HAND

36 Flexors of digits II and III – Passive stretch   **81**

37 Flexors of digits IV and V – Passive stretch   **83**

38 Flexors of digits II–V – Active whole hand opening   **85**

39 Flexors of digits II–V – Active extension of each digit   **87**

40 Interosseus muscles – Passive stretch   **89**

41 Interosseus muscles – Active extension of the first phalanx   **91**

THUMB

42 Long thumb flexor – Passive stretch   **93**

43 Long thumb flexor – Active long thumb extension   **95**

44 Short thumb flexor – Passive stretch   **97**

45 Short thumb flexor – Active short thumb extension   **99**

46 Opponens pollicis – Passive stretch   **101**

47 Long abductor of the thumb – Passive stretch   **103**

48 Opponens pollicis/Long abductor of the thumb –
   Active thumb deopposition/opposition   **105**

49 Adductor pollicis – Passive stretch   **107**

50 Adductor pollicis – Active short thumb abduction   **109**

APPENDIX

Personal log sheet – Lower limb   **111**

Personal log sheet – Upper limb   **114**

Neuroloco   **118**

Author biography

Jean-Michel Gracies, MD, PhD completed his residency in intensive care, neurorehabilitation, neurology, and acute stroke care at Hôpitaux de Paris, France and received his medical degree and doctorate in Neurophysiology from University of Paris VI. He completed a postdoctoral fellowship in the pathophysiology and therapy of spastic paresis at Prince of Wales Medical Research Institute in Sydney, Australia, and a fellowship in neurology/movement disorders at Mount Sinai Medical Center, New York. After working for 10 years as Attending and Clerkship Director in the Neurology department (Movement Disorders division) at Mount Sinai Medical Center, Professor Gracies took a position in 2007 as Professor and Chair in the Department of Rééducation Neurolocomotrice at Hôpitaux Universitaires Henri Mondor, Créteil, France. Professor Gracies has written over 200 original articles, book chapters, theses, reviews, and abstracts. He has served on the editorial board of *Journal of Neural Transmission* and is an ad hoc reviewer for *Brain, Experimental Brain research, Muscle and Nerve, Stroke, Movement Disorders, Journal of Neurology, Neuropsychiatry and Neurosurgery, Clinical Neuropharmacology, Clinical Neurophysiology, Archives of Physical Medicine and Rehabilitation, American Journal of Rehabilitation, Archives of Gerontology, and Geriatrics.*

Professor Gracies is a world-renowned expert on the neurorehabilitation of movement. As Head of the Department of Rééducation Neurolocomotrice at Hôpitaux Universitaires Henri Mondor, in Créteil, France, he is launching novel pathophysiological concepts, neurorehabilitation programs, and clinical research projects for syndromes such as spastic paresis, parkinsonian syndromes, tremors, peripheral facial palsies, falls in the elderly, and other movement disorders.

His main published contributions to date have been the design, naming, validation, and promotion of the Tardieu Scale for spastic paresis, which he later incorporated into a five-step Quantified Clinical Assessment of spastic paresis and the development of four Coefficients of Impairment in spastic paresis, the definition of the phenomenon of spastic cocontraction and its recognition as the primary disabling symptom in spastic paresis, and a technically antagonist-based and psychologically diary-based rehabilitation system in spastic paresis called the 'Guided Self-rehabilitation Contract'. Professor Gracies now promotes the use of similar diary-based moral contracts in other chronic disabling disorders. He is currently acting as the international coordinator of studies of spasticity using botulinum toxin. Professor Gracies lectures worldwide on the pathophysiology and treatment of spastic paresis, the neurorehabilitative treatment of Parkinson's disease, the treatment of tremors using botulinum toxin and motor strengthening, and programming methods for deep brain stimulation.

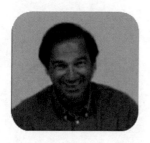

Dedicated to Lucian,
the patient who lit up the way

I am indebted to the following colleagues and collaborators who have helped with the illustrations and design of this work:

Inke-Marie ALBERTSEN, PhD
Marjolaine BAUDE, MD
Nicolas BAYLE, MD
Romain BLONDEL, MD
Caroline GAULT-COLAS, MD
Mouna GHEDIRA, PT, PhD
Emilie HUTIN, PhD
Hani KHAWAM
Catherine-Marie LOCHE, MD
Valentina MARDALE, MD
Maud PRADINES, PT, PhD
Tharaga SANTIAGO, PT

I would like to extend our sincere thanks to the patients who so graciously and generously agreed to participate in the demonstrations and photography sessions that helped create this manual of guided self-rehabilitation.

I am indebted to my dear colleagues Martina HOSKOVCOVÁ, MD and Ota GÁL, PT, PhD, from Charles University, Prague (CZ), for their valuable proof checking of the book.

Special thanks to Robert KAHOUD, MD, from the Mayo Clinic, Rochester (MN), for his precious edits from an English language perspective.

I am equally grateful to the entire team of the Department of Rééducation Neurolocomotrice of the Albert Chenevier – Henri Mondor University Hospitals.

Foreword

Understanding spastic paresis...

You probably opened this book because you are affected by a syndrome called spastic paresis, which is the consequence of, for example, a central nervous system disorder such as a stroke (cerebrovascular accident), traumatic brain or spinal cord injury, multiple sclerosis, or a tumor of the nervous system, conditions that may have occurred in childhood or in adulthood. This book is meant for you and for your therapists. The first reality to bear in mind (and that we will refer to at the end of this foreword) is that after these disorders or lesions, significant parts of your motor nervous system remain spared.

In spastic paresis, two problems coexist. The word 'paresis' means that when your brain sends the command to one of your muscles to contract, this order is incompletely received by the muscle. The word 'spastic' indicates that at the same time muscles cannot relax normally and have a tendency to be spontaneously overactive (muscle overactivity–spasticity), particularly if they are stretched too fast.

As it unfolds, the first cause of your functional difficulties, both in terms of timing and initial importance, is the paresis itself. Soon after, contracture of the soft tissues (for example, muscle shortening and stiffening) sets in and joins with paresis to act as a second cause of movement impairment. If nothing is done to oppose the contracture, it will continue to worsen. Muscle overactivity later adds a third cause of impairment. One form of muscle overactivity is called 'spastic co-contraction'; this is an involuntary activation of the muscle opposing the desired movement (antagonist), making that movement difficult (for example, contraction of the calf muscles when you want to raise your foot).

...and optimizing the function of the spared brain

The three fundamental processes responsible for your movement difficulties (paresis, soft tissue contracture, and muscle overactivity) do not equally affect the muscles on one side of the joint (agonist muscles) and the muscles on the other side of the joint (antagonists, producing movements that oppose the agonists). This asymmetry is responsible for force imbalances around joints, leading to both disfigurement at rest and difficulties when trying to move.

In this situation, your motor function becomes entangled in two vicious cycles, which we will need to break. First, muscle contracture and overactivity (spasticity) make each other worse, creating a harmful vicious cycle of contracture–spasticity–contracture, which affects your muscles. Second, you often tend to spare, or 'disuse', your paretic limb in everyday life; this disuse further weakens the command to this limb, participating in the second vicious cycle of paresis–disuse–paresis, which affects your brain.

Our approach is to avoid the use of systemic (oral or 'intrathecal') depressant drugs commonly used in spastic paresis – known as 'anti-spastic' drugs – whenever possible, because of their invariable, often insidious and therefore unrecognized adverse effects. Instead, following a systematic approach targeting one joint at a time, each specific mechanism of impairment (paresis, muscle contracture, or muscle overactivity) is treated focally, muscle by muscle, aiming to reestablish equilibrium among forces.

The program you are about to embark upon is an antagonist-based and diary-based rehabilitation system. For the most shortened and overactive muscles – which are antagonists to your attempted movements – a daily program of prolonged stretching – potentially in conjunction with focal injections of nerve blocking agents (botulinum toxin, for example) by your doctor – will help to lengthen and soften up the shortened and stiffened muscles to break the vicious cycle contracture–spasticity–contracture.

To improve voluntary command of your weaker muscles and reduce cocontraction of their antagonists, an intensive motor training program using unassisted large amplitude rapid alternating movements – or rapid alternating efforts when movements are not yet possible – will gradually increase brain command effectiveness. The goal here is to break the cycle paresis–disuse–paresis.

You and your therapist will target the most important muscles in your case and you will commit to a guided self-rehabilitation contract. 'Contract' here is not meant in the legal sense: this is a moral contract, in the sense of a mutual agreement between you and your therapist. In this contract, you are the champion who is in training to improve the performance of the part of your nervous system that remains spared. The therapist (eg, your physical therapist) can be viewed as your coach, just like a sports coach. For a long period (at least a year), you and your therapist will meet for longer but less frequent sessions than in traditional rehabilitation models. In these sessions, the two of you will select the most appropriate stretching and training exercises, ie, the most appropriate self-rehabilitation sheets in this manual. This selection may evolve with time, depending on your progress.

Each exercise should be difficult. If an exercise becomes easy with time, this means both that you have made progress and that this exercise has become inefficient for your brain; your therapist will adjust the difficulty level or change it for a more challenging one.

The terms of your contract include: (1) actively practicing the exercises prescribed in the sheets selected for you and; (2) keeping a written log/diary of your performance in this daily program. By following these terms, you will see your own hard work and dedication result in continued improvement, regardless of how much time has passed since your accident or the onset of your illness.

I now urge you to find and kindle that 'fire in your belly' motivation to achieve the required intensity, discipline, and consistency in your everyday work. It will pay off!

Introduction

Getting started with the guided self-rehabilitation contract

The following pages describe a series of stretching and training techniques that target the most frequently involved muscles (antagonists) in spastic paresis. Your therapist, whether a doctor, physical therapist, occupational therapist, psychomotor therapist, physical education teacher, or therapeutic nurse educator, will select, teach you, and prescribe the postures and exercises that are most needed in your particular case.

Each stretching or training technique can be practiced on your own at home, without the use of any expensive equipment. On each sheet you will find an explanation of the maneuver and its required duration on the left side, and an illustration on the right. We recommend preserving a cardiovascular rest period after each workout by alternating active training bouts – each one lasting 15–60 seconds – with stretching postures, to be maintained for 2–20 minutes.

During these exercises you may experience minor pain and discomfort related to muscle stretch or muscle use, which will dissipate when the activity is stopped. This is normal. If you have doubts about a particular exercise/training, or if the explanations are not sufficient, please seek advice from your therapist.

The color code will help you navigate the manual:

- blue colours in the title are used for passive stretch postures; and
- green colours in the title are used for active training exercises.

An important part of the contract is that you document your performance in the stretches and exercises you have executed every day. For this you may photocopy the logbook sheets at the end of the manual or create a logbook of your own. The exercises in this manual should be part of your daily routine and the time required for this self-rehabilitation should be integrated into your schedule.

The key words here are belief, intensity, and consistency. Have confidence in the capacity of a well-practiced stretching and training program to help you improve gradually over time, even if you will not always be aware of your progress.

Neuroloco

Reconquering Movement

www.neuroloco.org

(Non-profit association)

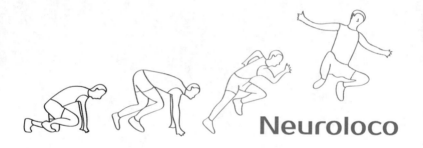

*Promoting Research in
Neurorehabilitation
and Orthopedic Rehabilitation*

Contact:
Hôpitaux Universitaires Henri Mondor
Service de Rééducation Neurolocomotrice
40 rue de Mesly, 94000 Créteil, France
Tél : +33-1-49-81-30-61
www.neuroloco.org

Lower limb anatomical review

Lower limb introduction

Anatomical review

Here are some simple definitions; the specific leg movements are illustrated in the photographs below:

- Hip flexion (green arrow) and extension (blue arrow) (Figure A)
- Hip abduction (green arrow) and adduction (blue arrow) (Figure B)
- Hip external rotation (green arrow) and internal rotation (blue arrow) (Figure C)
- Knee flexion (green arrow) and extension (blue arrow) (Figure D)
- Ankle dorsiflexion (green arrow) and plantar flexion (blue arrow) (Figure E)
- Swing phase of gait: this is the phase starting from when the foot takes off from the ground until it lands again.
- Stance phase of gait: this is the phase starting from when the foot lands on the ground until it leaves the ground again (Figure F).

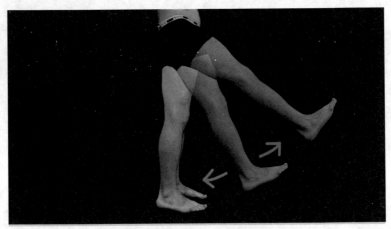

Figure A Hip flexion (green arrow) and hip extension (blue arrow).

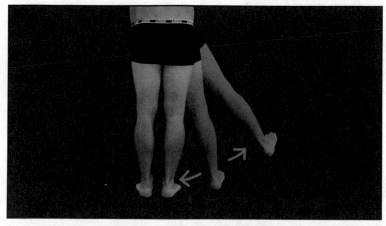

Figure B Hip abduction (green arrow) and hip adduction (blue arrow).

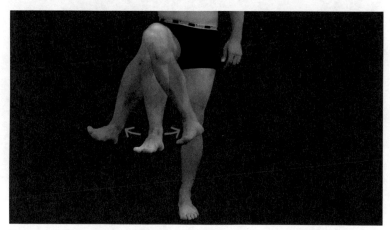

Figure C Hip external rotation (green arrow) and hip internal rotation (blue arrow).

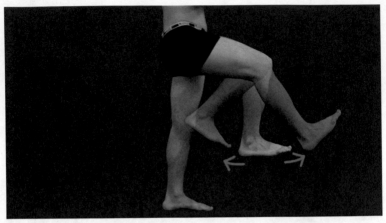

Figure D Knee flexion (green arrow) and knee extension (blue arrow).

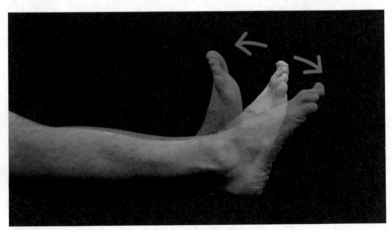

Figure E Ankle dorsiflexion (green arrow) and plantar flexion (blue arrow).

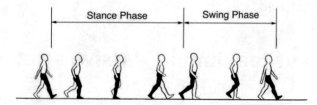

Figure F Stance phase and swing phase of gait. Published with kind permission of © The Queen's Printer for Ontario, 2016. All rights reserved.

HIP – Sheet 1

Gluteus maximus – Passive stretch

The gluteus maximus is the largest muscle in the body. It makes up most of the bulk of the buttock (Figure 1A) and is used to extend the hip, for example in standing up, running or walking fast.

If this muscle is hyperactive or too short, it impedes the hip flexion movement that should initiate the swing phase of gait.

The stretching posture is performed while lying on your back. The non-paretic hand grasps the knee, flexes, and pulls it towards the chest as close as possible; the non-paretic leg remains resting on the bed in full extension (Figure 1B). If possible, use the hand on the same side to pull the knee (Figure 1C). If need be, this position may be initiated and/or maintained with the help of another person (Figure 1D).

The stretching posture is performed correctly when you feel tension (not pain) in the gluteal region.

Remember to note in your personal log the total number of minutes that you perform this stretching posture each day.

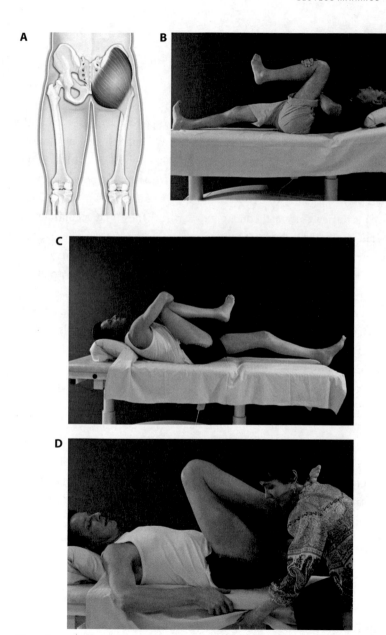

Figure 1

≥ -- minutes ≥ -- times per day

HIP – Sheet 2

Gluteus maximus – Active hip flexion, knee flexed

Active hip flexion is the one movement we use to start every walking step. Proper active hip flexion leads to passive knee flexion by inertia, which allows the foot to clear the ground. The movement of hip flexion is often incomplete or too slow in the setting of spastic paresis, which often plays a primary role in walking impairment.

This difficulty is partly due to excessive stiffness and cocontraction in gluteus maximus, hamstrings, and rectus femoris muscles. Resistance (stiffness) and cocontractions from gluteus maximus, hamstrings, and rectus femoris must therefore be reduced to improve amplitude, strength, and speed of active hip flexion at each step.

The best way to achieve this objective is to repeat sets of hip flexion exercises every day, trying to reach maximum amplitude and speed at each attempt.

This workout is performed while standing and holding onto a table, heavy object, or a bar to the side, possibly with your back against a wall. You must try and hold the paretic hand low, at hip height. Try to <u>lift the knee up</u> as high as possible to your hand and back down at each attempt (Figure 2A–B). Ideally, alternate sets of this exercise with gluteus maximus stretching postures (Sheet 1), as recommended by your therapist.

Note: For optimal hip flexion with the knee flexed, gluteus maximus, hamstrings, and rectus femoris muscles need to be sufficiently long and relaxed, which is why your therapist will ask you to stretch them (Sheets 1, 3, and 10) and your doctor may suggest injections of a neuromuscular blocker into these muscles.

Please note in your personal log the maximum number of active hip flexions (knee flexed) that you performed in --- seconds per set.

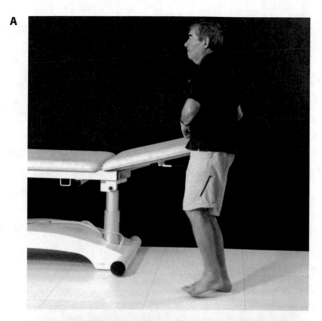

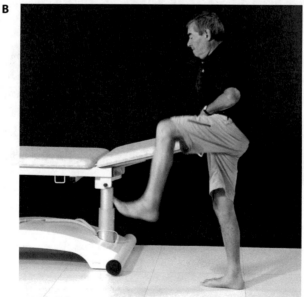

Figure 2

Maximum repetitions in -- seconds, -- times per day

HIP – Sheet 3

Hamstrings – Passive stretch

The hamstrings make up the bulk of the posterior compartment of the thigh. The semitendinosus muscle (internally) and biceps femoris (externally) are palpable under the skin and give its shape to the posterior thigh. The semimembranosus muscle is located most internally, next to the semitendinosus (Figure 3A). The hamstrings are used to extend the hip and flex the knee (for example in running, jumping, or walking fast). They are of little use in slow or medium speed walking. If these muscles are hyperactive or too short:

- They impede the hip flexion movement that should initiate the swing phase of gait.
- They also tend to prevent active knee extension in the middle of stance (vertical body propulsion) and re-extension at the end of swing to complete the step: at both times the knee stays excessively bent.

The stretching posture is maintained in a sitting position (Figure 3B and Figure 3C). You have placed the paretic foot on a chair in front of you (Figure 3B) so that the ankle and calf are supported. If placing the foot on a chair is too difficult, you may simply lay the leg straight on the floor (Figure 3C). The stretching posture will consist of the following:

- place your hand(s) on your knee to help keep the leg as straight as possible; and
- bend forward at the waist as much as possible, as if you were trying to flatten your chest against your leg (or to lay your head on your knee). Always keep the knee extended.

The stretching posture is performed correctly when you feel tension (not pain) behind the thigh.

> **Remember to note in your personal log the total number of minutes that you perform this stretching posture each day.**

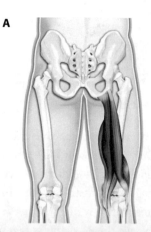

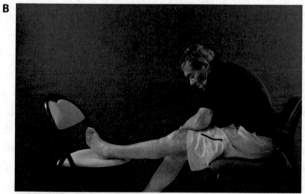

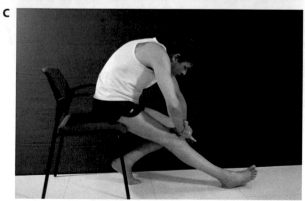

Figure 3

≥ -- minutes ≥ -- times per day

HIP – Sheet 4

Hamstrings – Active hip flexion, knee extended

The movement of active hip flexion with knee extended is not a frequently used movement in daily life (except for kicking a ball for example). However, the repeated exercise will help reduce resistance (stiffness) and cocontractions from the hamstrings, which is a muscle group that may impede hip flexion at each walking step.

The best way to achieve this objective is to repeat sets of hip flexion exercises with the knee extended every day, trying to reach maximum amplitude and speed at each attempt.

This workout is performed while standing and holding onto a table, a heavy object, or a bar to the side, possibly with your back against a wall. You should try to <u>lift your extended leg</u> as high as possible with each attempt (Figure 4A–B). Ideally, alternate sets of this exercise with hamstrings stretching postures (Sheet 3), as recommended by your therapist.

Note: For optimal hip flexion movements with the knee extended, hamstrings and gluteus maximus muscles need to be sufficiently long and relaxed, which is why your therapist will ask you to stretch them (Sheets 1 and 3) and your doctor may suggest injections of a neuromuscular blocker into these muscles.

Please note in your personal log the maximum number of active hip flexions (knee extended) that you achieved in the number of seconds per set.

A

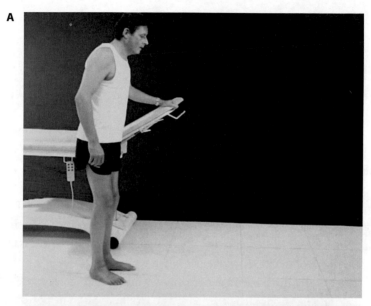

B

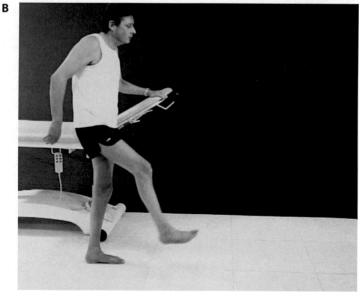

Figure 4

Maximum repetitions in -- seconds, -- times per day

HIP – Sheet 5

Hip flexor-adductors – Passive stretch

The hip flexor-adductor muscles are adductor brevis and adductor longus (Figure 5A). They are used to bring the thigh inward and help flex the hip during walking.

If these muscles are hyperactive or too short, they reduce the small spacing between the legs that is normally part of the swing phase. This can result in a 'scissoring' gait where the knees tend to collide when they pass each other: the leg in swing phase adducts too much by excessive involvement of the flexor-adductors in the hip flexion.

The stretching posture is performed while standing, legs straight and as far apart from each other as possible (Figure 5B). The posture is maintained with hands resting on a bar or a piece of furniture (table) in front of you.

To best stretch adductor brevis and longus, try to bring the pelvis as far forward as possible (Figure 5B).

The stretch is performed correctly when you feel tension (not pain) in the groin.

> **Remember to note in your personal log the total number of minutes that you perform this stretching posture each day.**

A

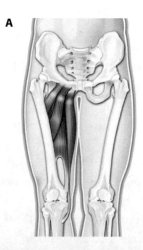

B

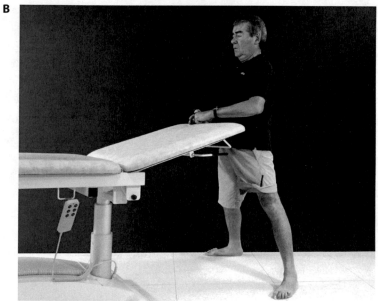

Figure 5

≥ -- minutes ≥ -- times per day

HIP – Sheet 6

Hip extensor-adductors –
Passive stretch

The hip extensor-adductor muscles are adductor magnus, gracilis, and pectineus (Figure 6A). They are used to bring the thigh inward and may stabilize the hip during walking. In addition, adductor gracilis tend to extend the hip and flex the knee. If these muscles are hyperactive or too short:

- They reduce the small spacing between the legs that is normally part of the swing phase. This can result in a 'scissoring' gait where the knees tend to collide when they pass each other or in an excessive inward movement of the foot before reaching the floor at the end of the swing phase, with then a reduced base of support.
- They also tend to hinder hip flexion at the beginning of the swing phase as well as knee re-extension at late swing phase.

The stretching posture is performed while sitting (Figure 6B). Place the paretic foot on a chair in front of you, so that the calf and foot are supported. Then try to lean towards the other knee instead of trying to reach the paretic knee (Figure 6C).

The stretching posture is performed correctly when you feel tension (not pain) in the inner thigh.

> **Remember to note in your personal log the total number of minutes that you perform this stretching posture each day.**

A
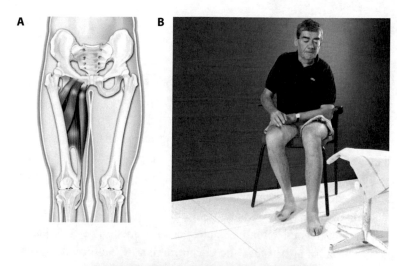

C
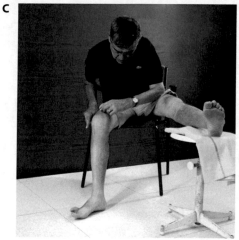

Figure 6

≥ -- minutes ≥ -- times per day

HIP – Sheet 7

Hip adductors – Active hip abduction

During gait, a small but sufficient bilateral hip abduction (slightly spreading legs apart) is required during each step to prevent the knee of the swinging leg from drifting inward and colliding with the other knee as it passes ahead of the supporting leg. Hip abduction is also necessary to keep balance in case of loss of equilibrium to one side.

This movement is often incomplete or restrained in case of spastic paresis because of stiffness and cocontraction in the hip adductors. Resistance (stiffness) and cocontraction from the hip adductors must therefore be reduced to facilitate active hip abduction with each step.

The best way to achieve this objective is to repeat sets of hip abduction exercises every day, trying to reach maximum amplitude and speed at each attempt.

This workout is performed while standing and holding on to a table, a heavy object, or a bar to the side, possibly leaning against a wall, and each time trying to lift the leg to the side as high as possible with the knee extended (Figure 7A–B). Ideally, alternate sets of this exercise with flexor-adductor and extensor-adductor stretching postures (Sheets 5 and 6), as recommended by your therapist.

Note: For optimal hip abduction the hamstrings and adductors need to be sufficiently long and relaxed, which is why your therapist will ask you to stretch them (Sheets 3, 5, and 6) and your doctor may suggest injections of a neuromuscular blocker into the extensor-adductor muscles.

Please note in your personal log the maximum number of hip abductions that you performed in --- seconds per set.

A

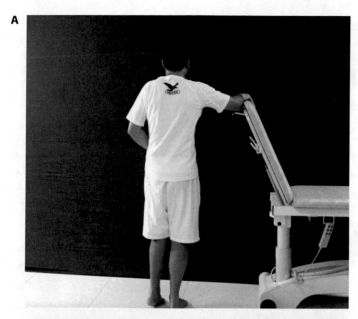

B

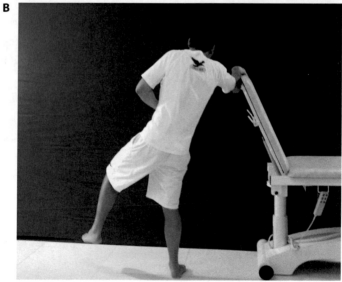

Figure 7

Maximum repetitions in -- seconds, -- times per day

HIP – Sheet 8

Hip internal rotators – Passive stretch

The hip internal rotator muscles are the gluteus minimus and the internal part of the gluteus medius (lateral part of hip), which form the bulk of the hip, and the tensor fascia lata (outer part of the thigh, Figure 8A). These muscles help bring the knee inward.

If these muscles are hyperactive or too short, they bring the knee and foot too far inward with respect to the walking axis, which alters balance in stance phase and causes difficulty flexing the hip in the swing phase.

The stretching posture may be performed while sitting (hip flexed at 90°) by placing the paretic foot on the opposite knee and pressing down firmly on the paretic knee <u>while bending forward</u> as much as possible (Figure 8B). The posture may also be maintained while lying down, <u>hip extended</u> with someone keeping the hip in external rotation (Figure 8C–D). The advantage of the latter posture is that the stretch is performed with the hip extended, which is closer to the natural walking positions and better stretches the tensor fascia lata.

The stretching posture is performed correctly when you feel tension (not pain) in the outer and upper thigh.

> **Remember to note in your personal log the total number of minutes that you perform this stretching posture each day.**

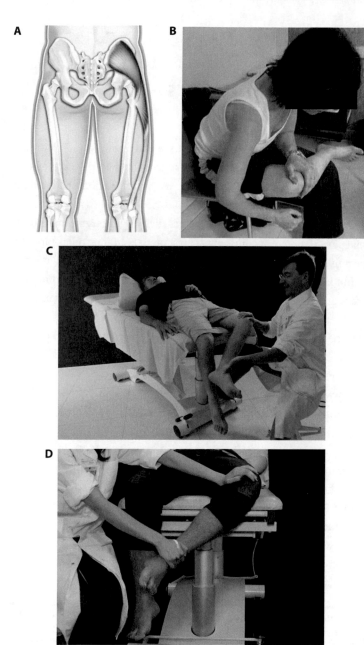

Figure 8

$\geq$ -- minutes $\geq$ -- times per day

HIP – Sheet 9

Hip internal rotators – Active hip external rotation

During gait, small but sufficient hip external rotation is required at each step to avoid internal rotation in swing phase in the case of short or overactive internal rotators. Indeed, when hip flexion or hip abduction is restrained, excessive recruitment of accessory hip flexors such as tensor fascia lata, accessory hip abductors such as gluteus minimus or the medial part of gluteus medius, may cause unwanted internal rotation, as these muscles are also internal rotators of the hip. The objective is thus to minimize resistance (stiffness) and cocontraction from hip internal rotators and improve amplitude, strength, and speed of external rotation movements.

The best way to achieve this objective is to repeat sets of hip external rotation exercises every day, trying to reach maximum amplitude and speed at each attempt.

This workout is performed <u>while lying down (hip extended)</u>, the leg dangling over the edge of the bed. You should try to <u>lift up the foot inward</u> as high as possible at each effort, which corresponds to hip external rotation (Figure 9A–B). Ideally, alternate sets of this exercise with hip internal rotator stretching postures (Sheet 8), as recommended by your therapist.

Note: For optimal hip external rotation, the medial part of gluteus medius and the gluteus minimus need to be sufficiently long and relaxed, which is why your therapist will ask you to stretch them (Sheet 8) and your doctor may suggest injections of a neuromuscular blocker into these muscles.

Please note in your personal log the maximum number of active hip external rotations performed in --- seconds per set.

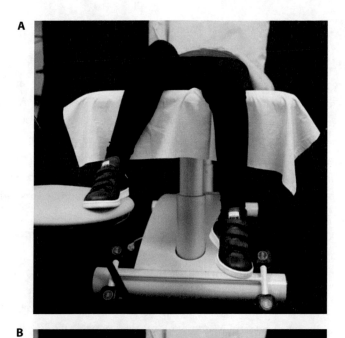

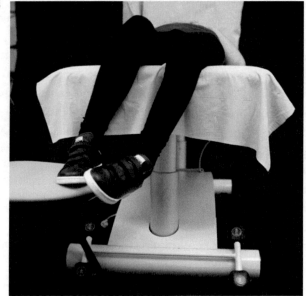

Figure 9

Maximum repetitions in -- seconds, -- times per day

KNEE – Sheet 10

Rectus femoris – Passive stretch

The rectus femoris muscle is located on the anterior aspect of the thigh. It is a part of the quadriceps, which extends the knee (Figure 10A). Among the four quadriceps heads, the rectus femoris muscle is the only one that is also used to flex the hip, which it does while extending the knee (this muscle is used for example to kick a ball, which requires combined hip flexion and knee extension). If this muscle is hyperactive or too short:

- It interferes with the passive knee flexion that normally accompanies and facilitates the first part of the swing phase of the step.
- It also hinders the passive hip extension that is required in the stance phase.
- If possible, the stretching posture may be performed while lying on your side: using the hand on the same side of the leg to be stretched, grasp the lower leg by the ankle and flex the knee by bringing the heel as close to the buttocks as possible while trying to pull the hip into extension (backward) as well. Keep the non-paretic leg resting on the bed (Figure 10B).
- If this action is impossible because of weakness or stiffness of the arm, this stretch can also be practiced alone lying on your back. You should bend your non-paretic leg, then have the paretic leg hanging from the side of the bed and stretch it pulling backwards with an elastic rope tied around your ankle, using your non-paretic arm (Figure 10C).
- The stretch can also be practiced while lying on your belly, the elastic rope pulled by your non-paretic arm to stretch the leg backwards (Figure 10D).
- If these actions are impossible, the stretching position can be initiated and/or maintained by another person (Figure 10E).

The stretching posture is performed correctly when you feel tension (not pain) in front of the thigh.

> **Remember to note in your personal log the total number of minutes that you perform this stretching posture each day.**

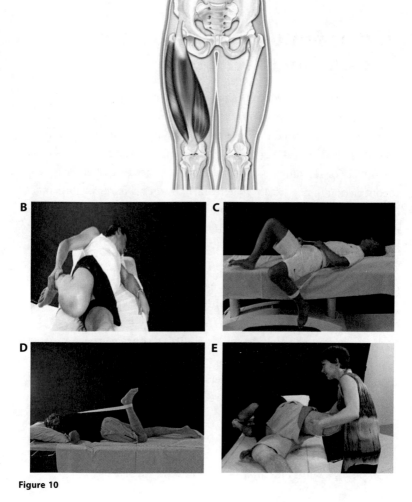

Figure 10

≥ -- minutes ≥ -- times per day

KNEE – Sheet 11

Rectus femoris – Active knee flexion, hip extended

Active knee flexion movement (kicking the foot backward) is of little use in daily life other than in running or brisk walking. However, quick passive knee flexion is required to clear the ground during the swing phase of each step or when walking up a flight of stairs. This movement is often incomplete or restrained with spastic paresis, because of stiffness and cocontraction in quadriceps, particularly in rectus femoris. Resistance (stiffness) and cocontractions from rectus femoris must therefore be reduced to facilitate passive knee flexion with each step.

The best way to achieve this objective is to repeat sets of active knee flexion exercises backwards in standing position, trying to reach maximum amplitude and speed at each attempt.

This workout is performed while standing next to a table, heavy object or a bar, trying to raise your foot as high as possible towards your back. This means bringing the thigh and <u>lifting your knee backward </u>and not forward, as if you were trying to hit your buttocks with your heel (Figure 11A–B). Ideally, alternate sets of this exercise with rectus femoris stretching postures (Sheet 10), as recommended by your therapist.

Note: For an optimal active knee flexion movement the quadriceps needs to be sufficiently long and relaxed, which is why your therapist will ask you to stretch it (Sheet 10 and 12) and your doctor may suggest injections of a neuromuscular blocker into this muscle.

Please note in your personal log the maximum number of active knee flexions, hip extended that you performed in --- seconds per set.

A

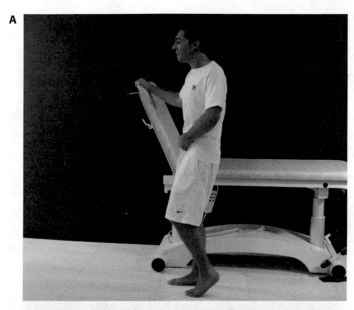

B

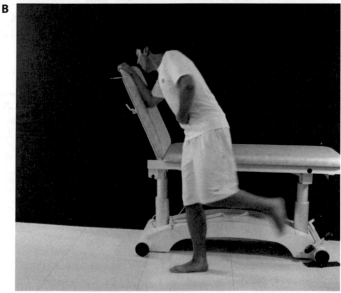

Figure 11

Maximum repetitions in -- seconds, -- times per day

KNEE – Sheet 12

Vastus muscles – Passive stretch

The vastus muscles (vastus intermedius, vastus lateralis, and vastus medialis) are located on the anterior and lateral aspects of the thigh (Figure 12A). Surrounding the rectus femoris, the three vastus muscles make up the whole quadriceps, which is the bulk of the front compartment of the thigh. The three vastus muscles only extend the knee, with no direct action on the hip.

If these muscles are hyperactive or too short, they interfere with the passive knee flexion that normally accompanies and facilitates the first part of the swing phase of the step.

If possible, **the stretching posture** may be performed while kneeling on a mat: you may kneel while using the support of a chair next to you (Figure 12B). Place your feet as much apart from each other as possible and then bring your buttocks as low as possible between your feet (Figure 12C).

The stretching posture is performed correctly when you feel tension (not pain) in front and on the sides of the thigh.

Remember to note in your personal log the total number of minutes that you perform this stretching posture each day.

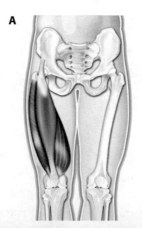

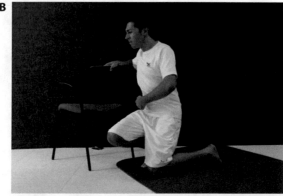

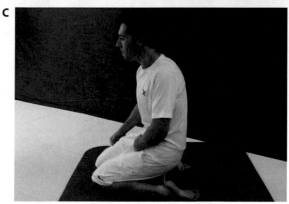

Figure 12

≥ -- minutes ≥ -- times per day

KNEE – Sheet 13

Vastus muscles – Active knee flexion, hip flexed

Active knee flexion movement (kicking the foot backward) with the hip flexed (seated for example) is of little use in daily life. However, quick passive knee flexion is required to clear the ground during the swing phase of each step or when walking up a flight of stairs. This movement is often incomplete or restrained with spastic paresis because of stiffness and cocontraction in quadriceps. Resistance (stiffness) and cocontractions from vastus muscles must therefore be reduced to facilitate passive knee flexion with each step.

The best way to achieve this objective is to repeat sets of active knee flexion exercises from a high-seated position, trying to reach maximum amplitude and speed at each attempt, every day.

This workout is performed while sitting on a high chair, trying to bring your foot backward as high as possible, as if you were trying to hit your buttocks with your heel (Figure 13A–B). Ideally, alternate sets of this exercise with vastus muscles stretching postures (Sheet 12), as recommended by your therapist.

Note: For an optimal active knee flexion movement with hip flexed, the vastus muscles needs to be sufficiently long and relaxed, which is why your therapist will ask you to stretch them (Sheet 12) and your doctor may suggest injections of a neuromuscular blocker into these muscles.

> **Please note in your personal log the maximum number of active knee flexions, hip flexed that you performed in --- seconds per set.**

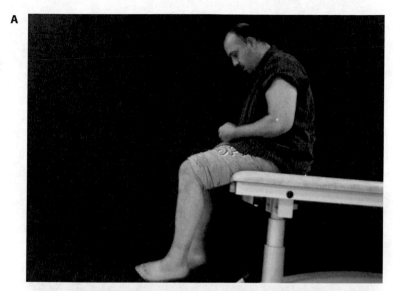

A

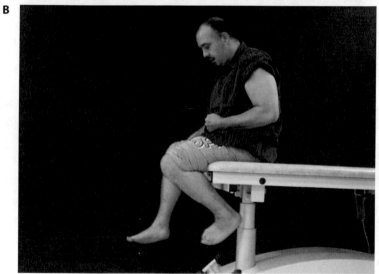

B

Figure 13

Maximum repetitions in -- seconds, -- times per day

ANKLE – Sheet 14

Soleus – Passive stretch

The soleus is a large muscle that makes up most of the bulk of the calf (Figure 14A). It is the main component of the triceps surae, which extends the ankle (plantar flexion), with the knee either extended or flexed. The soleus muscle is used to propel the whole body forward at the end of the stance phase in a brisk walk or run, or during jumping. It is of little use in slow or medium speed walking. If this muscle is hyperactive or too short:

- It causes an excessive extension of the knee when the foot is on the ground at stance phase ('knee snapping back').
- It then also blocks passive ankle dorsiflexion, preventing the body from pivoting forward around the ankle, which is needed for the other leg to step forward.
- In the swing phase, it prevents proper lifting of the foot, which is necessary to avoid tripping on the ground.

The stretching posture is performed using your body weight while standing. You will need a wedge (angle of about 20°) and a bathroom scale. Place the wedge up on the scale (Figure 14B). While holding onto a table, heavy object, or a bar, step up on the wedge with your paretic ankle (Figure 14C). <u>While keeping your knee bent</u> as much as you can (Figure 14D) lean as far forward as possible.

The stretching posture is performed correctly when you feel tension (not pain) in the mid or lower calf. The posture will also stretch additional plantar flexors, including the peroneus longus and the long toe flexor muscles (flexor hallucis longus and flexor digitorum longus) if the toes lay on the wedge and not outside.

> **Remember to note in your personal log the total number of minutes that you perform this stretching posture each day.**

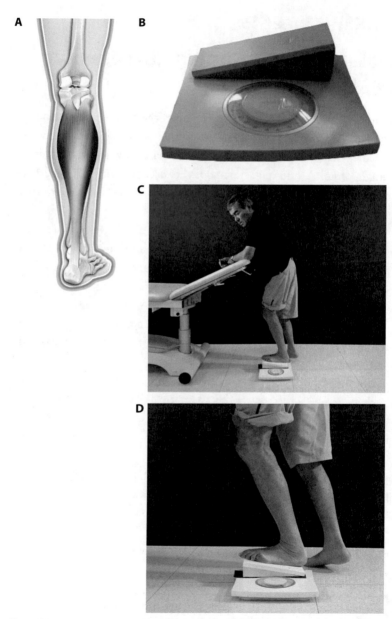

Figure 14

≥ -- minutes ≥ -- times per day

ANKLE – Sheet 15

Soleus – Active ankle dorsiflexion, seated

Active ankle dorsiflexion (raising the tip of the foot off the ground) in the position knee flexed is a movement that is used at each step when the knee flexes properly during the swing phase, or when walking down a flight of stairs. If this movement does not occur or is insufficient, there is a risk of tripping on the ground with the tip of the foot at every step, especially on uneven ground or in stairs.

This movement is often incomplete or restrained in the case of spastic paresis because of stiffness and cocontraction in the plantar flexors, particularly in soleus. Resistance (stiffness) and cocontractions from soleus must therefore be reduced to facilitate active ankle dorsiflexion with each step.

The best way to achieve this objective is to repeat sets of ankle dorsiflexion exercises in a sitting position every day, trying to reach maximum amplitude and speed at each attempt.

This workout is performed in a sitting position <u>with the knee at a right angle</u> if possible, each time trying to <u>lift the ball of your foot</u> as high off the ground as possible, as you would to the beat of a song (Figure 15A–C). Ideally, alternate sets of this exercise with soleus stretching postures (Sheet 14), as recommended by your therapist.

Note: For optimal active ankle dorsiflexion movement in the sitting position the soleus, long toe flexor muscles (flexor hallucis longus and flexor digitorum longus), and peroneus longus muscles need to be sufficiently long and relaxed, which is why your therapist will ask you to stretch them (Sheet 14) and your doctor may suggest injections of a neuromuscular blocker into these muscles.

> **Please note in your personal log the maximum number of active ankle dorsiflexions that you performed in --- seconds per set.**

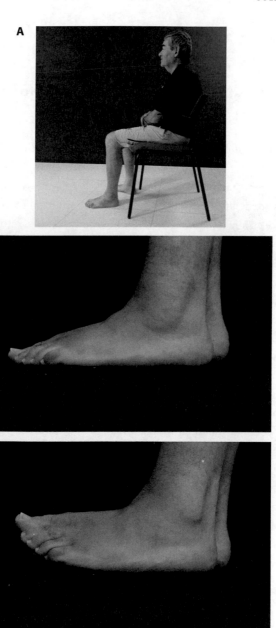

Figure 15

Maximum repetitions in -- seconds, -- times per day

ANKLE – Sheet 16

Gastrocnemius (medial and lateral) – Passive stretch

The gastrocnemius muscles are two superficial muscles (medial and lateral) that wrap the soleus in the calf (Figure 16A). They contribute to the triceps surae, which extends the ankle (plantar flexion), although the gastrocnemius muscles only extend the ankle when the knee is in extension. They serve to propel the whole body forward into a brisk walk or run. They are of little use in slow or medium speed walking. If these muscles are hyperactive or too short:

- They prevent the body from pivoting forward around the supporting foot at stance phase.
- They prevent knee extension in the middle of the stance phase and knee re-extension at the end of the swing phase: the knee then stays too flexed.
- During the swing phase, they prevent proper lifting of the foot, which is necessary to avoid tripping on the ground.

The stretching posture is performed <u>while standing, knee extended,</u> having set your foot on a wedge (angle of about 20°) itself placed on a bathroom scale, as with the soleus stretch (Sheet 14). Hold on to a table, a heavy object, or a bar in front of you and <u>bend the body</u> as far forward as possible, keeping your knee straight (Figure 16B–C).

The stretching posture is performed correctly when you feel tension (not pain) in the upper calf. The posture will also stretch additional plantar flexors, including the peroneus longus and the long toe flexor muscles (flexor hallucis longus and flexor digitorum longus) if the toes lay on the wedge and not outside.

Remember to note in your personal log the total number of minutes that you perform this stretching posture each day.

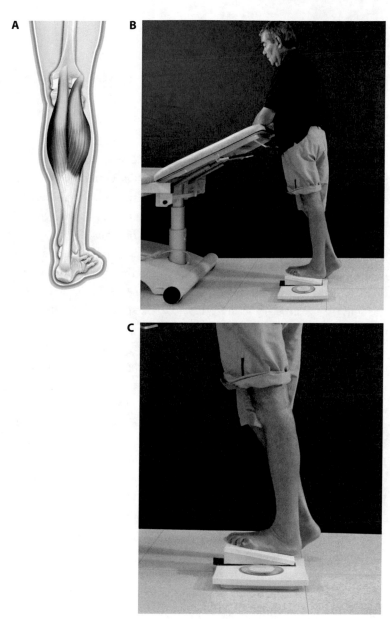

Figure 16

≥ -- minutes ≥ -- times per day

ANKLE – Sheet 17

Gastrocnemius – Active ankle dorsiflexion, standing

Active ankle dorsiflexion (raising the tip of the foot off the ground) with the knee extended is a movement that is required at each step when the knee does not flex well during the swing phase – a common situation in spastic paresis – or when walking up a flight of stairs. If this movement does not occur or is insufficient, there is a risk of tripping on the ground with every step, especially on uneven ground or on stairs.

This movement is often incomplete or restrained in the case of spastic paresis because of stiffness and cocontraction in the plantar flexors, particularly in the gastrocnemius muscles. Resistance (stiffness) and cocontractions from gastrocnemius must therefore be reduced to facilitate active ankle dorsiflexion with each step.

The best way to achieve this objective is to repeat series of ankle dorsiflexion exercises in a standing position every day, trying to reach maximum amplitude and speed at each attempt.

This workout is performed while standing next to a table, a heavy object, or a bar, possibly leaning against a wall. You need to try to <u>lift the ball of your foot</u> as high off the ground as possible, the <u>knee remaining extended</u> (Figure 17A–B). Ideally, alternate sets of this exercise with gastrocnemius stretching postures (Sheet 16), as recommended by your therapist.

This exercise can be frustrating as it is sometimes difficult to see the foot move when attempting to lift it off; sometimes the foot even moves down instead of up (Figure 17B bottom right). Remember however, that what matters first to your nervous system recovery is the repeated **effort** of transmitting a difficult order along the motor command pathways, not necessarily the gratification of seeing the foot actually move in the right direction.

Note: For optimal active ankle dorsiflexion movement in the standing position the gastrocnemius, soleus, long toe flexors (flexor hallucis longus and flexor digitorum longus), and peroneus longus need to be sufficiently long and relaxed, which is why your therapist asked you to stretch them (Sheet 14 and Sheet 16) and your doctor may suggest injections of a neuromuscular blocker into these muscles.

> **Please note in your personal log the maximum number of active ankle dorsiflexions that you performed in --- seconds per set.**

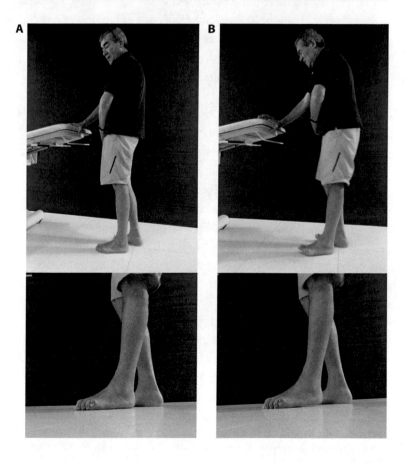

Figure 17

Maximum repetitions in -- seconds, -- times per day

LOWER LIMB FUNCTIONAL EXERCISES – Sheet 18

Sit-to-stand

Standing up is a prerequisite to human ambulation. The movement to stand up involves muscles that are also fundamental to standing balance (spine extensors, gluteus maximus and medius, knee extensors, and plantar flexors). If these muscles are weak, poorly balanced between either side of the body, or if resistance from knee or hip flexors is excessive, standing up and balance are compromised, with an increased risk of falling and difficulty getting up.

The sit-to-stand movement is often difficult in paraparesis and imbalanced in the case of hemiparesis or asymmetrical paraparesis, with a tendency to excessively load the body weight on the better leg. This behavior promotes disuse of the more paretic leg, further antagonizing neurological recovery (see Foreword). We must therefore improve its symmetry, strength, and speed.

The best way to achieve this objective is to repeat sets of sit-to-stand exercises at maximum speed every day, using a technique allowing optimal loading of the weaker leg (Figure 18A–C).

This workout is performed from a normal height chair, using a starting foot position in which <u>the more paretic foot is placed slightly **behind** the other foot</u> on the ground. You should try to stand up off the chair completely (so that the whole body becomes straight) followed by sitting back down. Repeat as fast as possible.

Note: For optimal sit-to-stand movements, the hamstrings need to be sufficiently long and relaxed, which is why your therapist will ask you to stretch them (Sheet 3) and your doctor may suggest injections of a neuromuscular blocker into these muscles.

Please note in your personal log the maximum number of sit-to-stand and stand-to-sit movements performed in --- seconds per set.

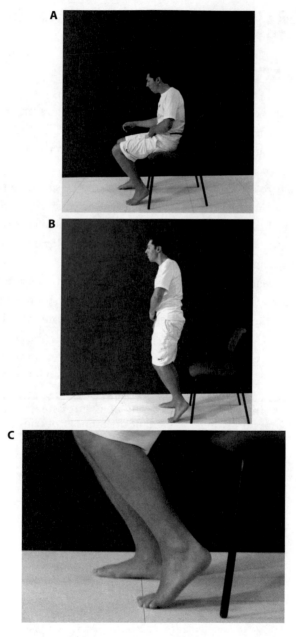

Figure 18

Maximum repetitions in -- seconds, -- times per day

LOWER LIMB FUNCTIONAL EXERCISES – Sheet 19

Long stride walking

Stride length is often reduced in the case of paresis. However, the ability to walk with long steps is associated with a better balance, lesser energy consumption, and a better style of natural walking. You must therefore work on increasing the stride length.

One way to achieve this objective is to walk the same pre-selected distance several times every day, while counting your steps and trying to cover the distance with the least number of steps possible. Every day you will try to beat your record of the smallest possible number of steps to cover the same distance (Figure 19A–B).

When it seems that you cannot beat your own record after several tries, you will double the distance and restart the program on the new distance.

Note: For the longest possible steps, the plantar flexors and the hamstrings need to be sufficiently long and relaxed, which is why your therapist will ask you to stretch them (Sheets 3, 14, and 16) and your doctor may suggest injections of a neuromuscular blocker into these muscles.

> **Please note in your personal log the number of steps taken to reach the target distance in each of the number of tries.**

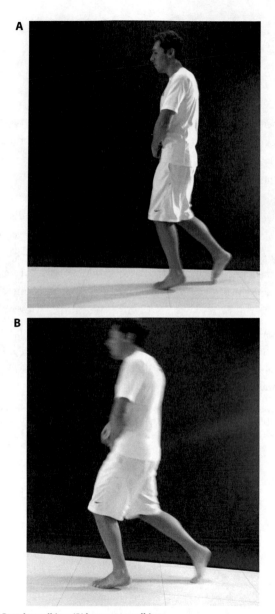

Figure 19 (A) Regular walking; (B) large step walking.

Each day walk the target distance --- times with as few steps as possible

LOWER LIMB FUNCTIONAL EXERCISES – Sheet 20

Fast walking

Walking speed is often reduced in the case of paresis. The practice of fast walking has been shown to facilitate gait improvement and achieving faster gait has been associated with increased ambulation in daily life. You must therefore work on increasing walking speed.

One way to achieve this objective is to walk the same pre-selected distance several times every day, while trying to cover the distance in as little time as possible. Every day you will try to beat your record of the shortest duration to cover the same distance (Figure 20A–B).

When it seems that you cannot beat your own record after several tries, you will double the distance and restart the program on the new distance.

Note: For the fastest possible walk, the plantar flexors, gluteus maximus, hamstrings, and quadriceps need to be sufficiently long and relaxed, which is why your therapist will ask you to stretch them (Sheets 1, 3, 10, 12, 14, and 16) and your doctor may suggest injections of a neuromuscular blocker into these muscles.

> **Please note in your personal log the number of seconds taken to reach the target distance in each of the number of tries.**

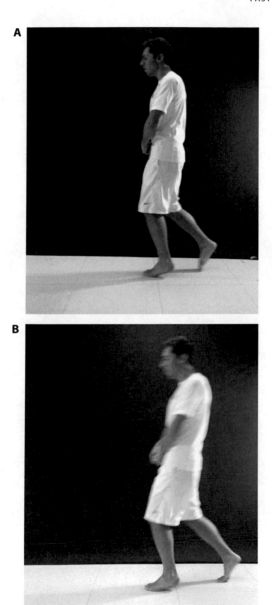

Figure 20 (A) Regular walking; (B) fast walking.

Each day walk the target distance --- times as fast as possible

Upper limb anatomical review

Upper limb introduction

Anatomical review

Here are some simple definitions; the specific arm movements are illustrated in the photographs below:

- Shoulder abduction (green arrow) and adduction (blue arrow) (Figure G)
- Shoulder flexion (green arrow) and extension (blue arrow) (Figure H)
- Shoulder external (green arrow) and internal rotation (blue arrow) (Figure I)
- Elbow extension (green arrow) and flexion (blue arrow) (Figure J)
- Elbow supination (green arrow) and pronation (blue arrow) (Figure K)
- Wrist extension (green arrow) and flexion (blue arrow) (Figure L)
- Finger extension (green arrow) and flexion (blue arrow) (Figure M)
- As per convention the fingers are numbered I to V (Figure N).

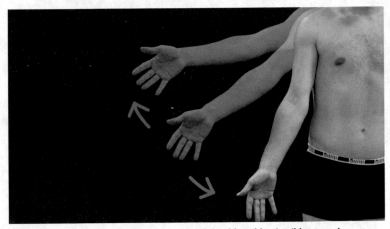

Figure G Shoulder abduction (green arrow) and shoulder adduction (blue arrow).

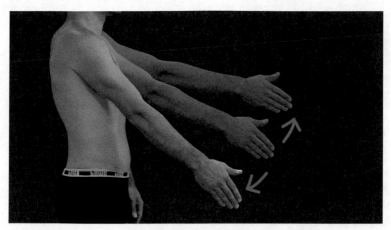

Figure H Shoulder flexion (green arrow) and shoulder extension (blue arrow).

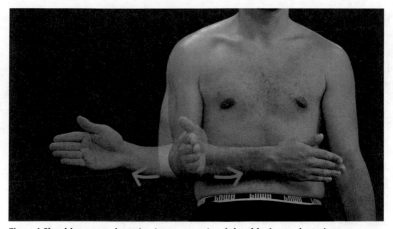

Figure I Shoulder external rotation (green arrow) and shoulder internal rotation (blue arrow).

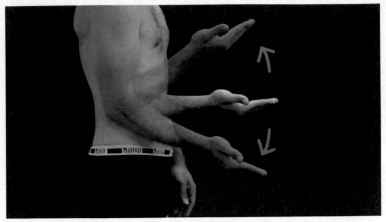

Figure J Elbow extension (green arrow) and elbow flexion (blue arrow).

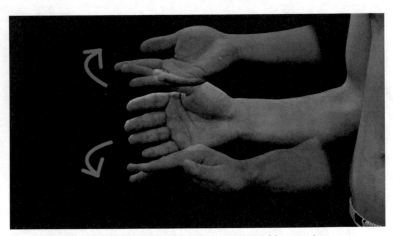

Figure K Elbow supination (green arrow) and elbow pronation (blue arrow).

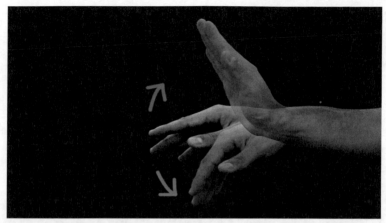

Figure L Wrist extension (green arrow) and wrist flexion (blue arrow).

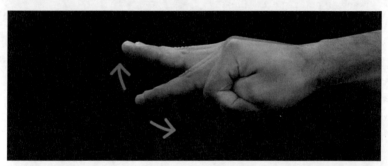

Figure M Finger extension (green arrow) and finger flexion (blue arrow).

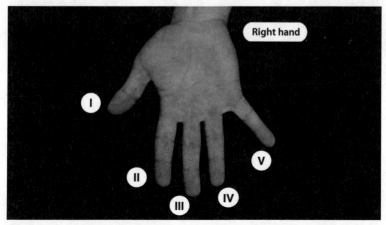

Figure N As per convention the fingers are numbered I to V as shown in the figure.

SHOULDER – Sheet 21

Pectoralis major – Passive stretch

The pectoralis major muscle makes up the anterior wall of the axilla (Figure 21A). It is easily palpable under the skin. This muscle is used to bring the arm back toward the body from outstretched positions to the front, the back or the side. If this muscle is overactive or too short:

- It impedes the shoulder abduction movement ie, stretching the arm out to the side to reach for support in case of imbalance
- It impedes shoulder flexion ie, stretching the arm out to the front to reach an object placed ahead.

Reducing the stiffness of this muscle by sufficient stretching often plays a crucial part in the functional recovery of the arm in spastic paresis.

The stretching posture is performed <u>in the sitting position</u>, for example on a couch with the paretic arm laid backward around the shoulders of another person or on top of the back rest (using a support system to keep the posture if possible, for example holding on to a stable object with your hand; Figure 21B–D).

Optimal stretching is achieved when you turn your head and trunk to the opposite side, while keeping your arm in position.

This stretch is performed properly when you feel tension (not pain) in the anterior wall of the axilla.

Remember to note in your personal log the total number of minutes that you perform this stretching posture each day.

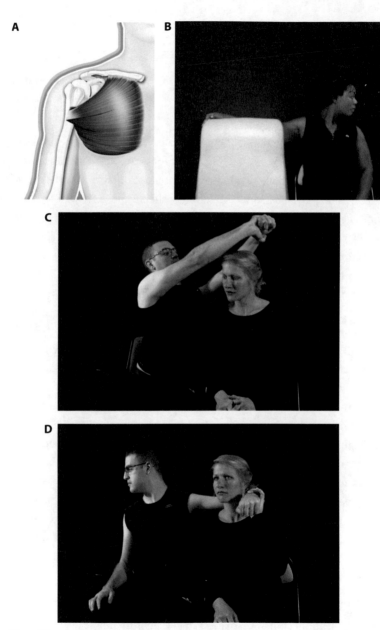

Figure 21

$\geq$ -- minutes $\geq$ -- times per day

SHOULDER – Sheet 22

Pectoralis major – Active shoulder abduction

Active shoulder abduction is the movement you use to grasp an object placed up high and to the side (on a shelf for example). This movement imposes stretch on shoulder adductors, latissimus dorsi, pectoralis major, and teres major in particular, which may then oppose shoulder abduction. The objective is thus to diminish the resistances coming from these shoulder adductors to improve amplitude, strength, and speed of shoulder abduction movements.

The best way to achieve this objective is to repeat sets of shoulder abduction exercises of maximum amplitude and speed every day.

This workout is best practiced while standing <u>with your side up against a wall</u> – or seated if the standing position is impossible. Mark the wall with a target at the maximum height you can reach with your hand outstretched to the side. The distance between the wall and the foot nearest to it should be the maximum distance that still allows you to barely reach the target. The hand movement starts from the hip, then up to the target and back, and is repeated as many times as possible in each set (Figure 22A–B). Ideally, alternate sets of this exercise with pectoralis major stretching postures (Sheet 21), as recommended by your therapist.

Note: For optimal shoulder abduction movement the latissimus dorsi, pectoralis major, and teres major muscles need to be long and well relaxed, which is why your therapist will ask you to stretch them (Sheets 21 and 23) and your doctor may suggest injections into these muscles with a neuromuscular blocker.

Please note in your personal log the maximum number of active shoulder abductions performed in --- seconds per set.

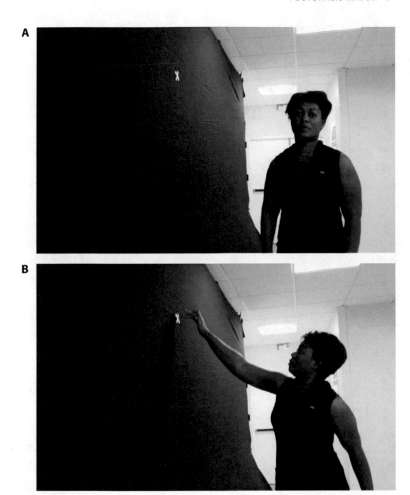

Figure 22

Maximum repetitions in -- seconds, -- times per day

SHOULDER – Sheet 23

Latissimus dorsi and long head of triceps – Passive stretch

The latissimus dorsi and the long head of triceps muscles make up the bulk of the posterior wall of the axilla (Figure 23A). They join the pectoralis major to help bring the arm back toward the body from outstretched positions to the front or side. The latissimus dorsi is the most involved muscle when bringing the arm backward (shoulder extension), which is used for example when holding onto a ramp or in rowing. The long head of triceps is a double extensor of both the shoulder and the elbow, which allows the extended arm to move backwards. If these muscles are overactive or too short:

- They impede the shoulder flexion movement, that is to say, the upward and forward movement of the arm to reach for an object in front of you.
- The long head of triceps especially hinders shoulder flexion with a flexed or semi-flexed elbow, which is a natural position when you begin to reach for an object placed high in front of you (eg, on a shelf).

Depending on the extensibility of the muscles, **the stretching posture** can be accomplished standing facing a wall and <u>placing the fully flexed elbow as high as possible</u> on the wall (Figure 23B). If this remains too difficult, the stretching posture can be achieved while sitting at a table and placing the flexed elbow as high as possible, for example on a stack of books in front of you (Figure 23C–D).

This stretch is performed properly when you feel tension (not pain) in the posterior wall of the axilla or the back of the upper arm.

Remember to note in your personal log the total number of minutes that you perform this stretching posture each day.

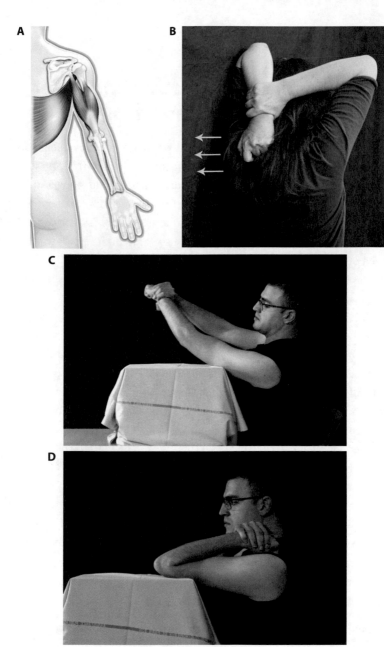

Figure 23

≥ -- minutes ≥ -- times per day

SHOULDER – Sheet 24

Latissimus dorsi – Active shoulder flexion, elbow extended

Active shoulder flexion with your elbow extended is the movement you use every time you grasp an object placed far and high in front of you. This movement stretches the shoulder extensors, latissimus dorsi, pectoralis major, teres major, and rhomboids in particular, which may then oppose shoulder flexion. The objective is thus to diminish the resistance coming from these shoulder extensors to improve the amplitude, strength, and speed of shoulder flexion movements with the elbow extended.

The best way to achieve this objective is to repeat sets of shoulder flexion exercises of maximum amplitude and speed every day.

This workout is best done <u>while standing in front of the wall</u> – or seated if the standing position is impossible – on which a target has been marked at the maximum height reachable by your hand. Similarly, the distance between the feet and the wall should be the maximum distance that still allows you to barely reach the target. The hand movement starts from the hip, up to the target and back, and is repeated as many times as possible during each set. <u>Keep your elbow straight</u> during the exercise (Figure 24A–B). Ideally, alternate sets of this exercise with the pectoralis major or the long head of triceps stretching postures (Sheets 21 and 23), as recommended by your therapist.

Note: For optimal shoulder flexion movement with the elbow extended, the latissimus dorsi, pectoralis major, teres major, and rhomboid muscles need to be long and well relaxed, which is why your therapist will ask you to stretch them (Sheets 21 and 23) and your doctor may suggest injections into these muscles with a neuromuscular blocker.

Please note in your personal log the maximum number of active shoulder flexions elbow extended performed in --- seconds per set.

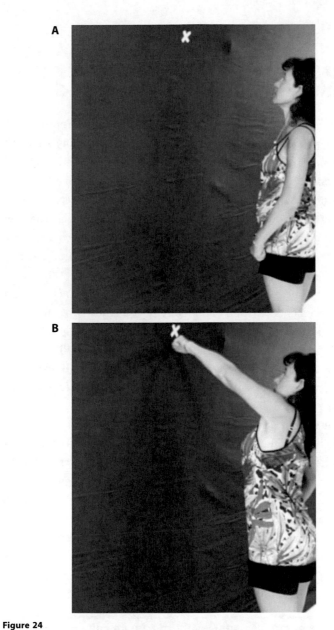

Figure 24

Maximum repetitions in -- seconds, -- times per day

SHOULDER – Sheet 25

Long head of triceps – Active shoulder flexion, elbow flexed

Active shoulder flexion with the elbow completely flexed is used when scratching your neck, combing your hair, or when reaching an object placed up high but close in front of you. Even if the object is high and far, it is natural to begin the movement with a slightly flexed elbow. This flexed position of the elbow stretches the long head of triceps, a double extensor of the shoulder and the elbow, which may then oppose shoulder flexion. The objective is thus to diminish the resistances coming from the long head of triceps to improve amplitude, strength, and speed of shoulder flexion movements with the elbow flexed.

The best way to achieve this objective is to repeat sets of shoulder flexion movements – with a completely flexed elbow – of maximum amplitude and speed every day.

This workout is best done while standing in front of a wall – or seated if the standing position is impossible – on which a target has been marked at the maximum height reachable by your elbow. You start by fully bending your elbow and pinning your hand to your neck (if necessary, use your other hand to keep it there). The distance between your feet and the wall should be the maximum distance that still allows your elbow to barely reach the target. Then, lift up your flexed elbow as high as possible toward the target, and bring it back down after each repetition (Figure 25A–B). Ideally, alternate sets of this exercise with the long head of triceps stretching postures (Sheet 23), as recommended by your therapist.

Note: For optimal shoulder flexion movement with the elbow flexed, the long head of triceps needs to be long and well relaxed, which is why your therapist will ask you to stretch it (Sheet 23) and your doctor may suggest injections into this muscle with a neuromuscular blocker.

Please note in your personal log the maximum number of active shoulder flexions elbow flexed performed in --- seconds per set.

A

B

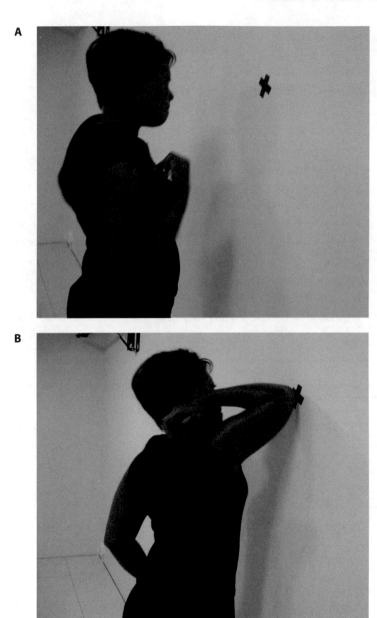

Figure 25

Maximum repetitions in -- seconds, -- times per day

SHOULDER – Sheet 26

Sub-scapularis – Passive stretch

The sub-scapularis is a shoulder internal rotator located deep in the posterior wall of the axilla (Figure 26A). This muscle joins teres major, pectoralis major, and latissimus dorsi to bring the hand inward to the belly.

If this muscle is overactive or too short, it hinders the external rotation of the shoulder that is involved in reaching movements of the arm towards close objects in front and to the side of you.

This stretching posture can be achieved while sitting: place the flexed elbow close to the body with the one hand grabbing a bar or a piece of furniture while the other hand keeps the elbow inward by pulling it close to the body (Figure 26B–C).

The stretch is performed properly when you feel tension (not pain) deep in the shoulder.

Remember to note in your personal log the total number of minutes that you perform this stretching posture each day.

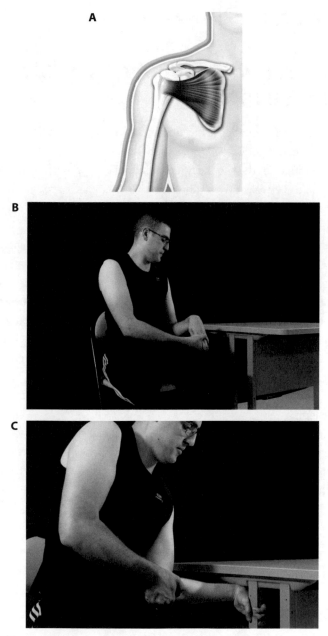

Figure 26

≥ -- minutes ≥ -- times per day

SHOULDER – Sheet 27

Sub-scapularis – Active shoulder external rotation

Shoulder external rotation is the movement we use to grasp objects close to the side of our bodies. This movement stretches the subscapularis, an internal rotator of the shoulder, which may then oppose external rotation. The objective is thus to diminish the resistance coming from the subscapularis to improve the amplitude, strength, and speed of external rotation at the shoulder.

The best way to achieve this objective is to repeat sets of shoulder external rotation exercises of maximum amplitude and speed every day.

This workout is best done while sitting, having placed a chair against the wall at an angle with the wall corresponding to the maximum opening angle of the forearm. The movements are carried out <u>while keeping your elbow close to your body</u> as if it were glued to it. The hand movement starts from the belly outward to touch the wall and back and is repeated with each effort (Figure 27A–D). Ideally, alternate sets of this exercise with subscapularis stretching postures (Sheet 26), as recommended by your therapist.

Note: For optimal shoulder external rotation movement, the subscapularis need to be long and well relaxed, which is why your therapist will ask you to stretch it (Sheet 26) and your doctor may suggest injections into this muscle with a neuromuscular blocker.

> **Please note in your personal log the maximum number of active shoulder external rotations performed in --- seconds per set.**

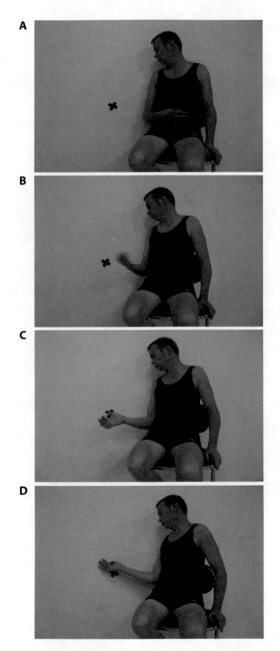

Figure 27

Maximum repetitions in -- seconds, -- times per day

ELBOW – Sheet 28

Elbow flexors – Passive stretch

The elbow flexor muscles form the bulk of the front compartment of the arm. The three most powerful flexor muscles are the biceps, which are superficial and especially active when bending the elbow with the palm up (supination); the brachialis, which lies deep and is especially active when bending the elbow with the palm down (pronation); and the brachioradialis, located in the outer part of the forearm, which is most active when bending the elbow with the hand in the neutral position (Figure 28A). The biceps are also strong supinators, which we will review in the supination training exercises. If these muscles are overactive or too short, they impede elbow extension, used when trying to reach an object placed in front of you.

The stretching posture is performed in a sitting position <u>while your legs are crossed and you bend forward at the waist</u>. Place your elbow on the opposite knee. Using your other hand, grab your wrist and extend your elbow, <u>twisting your forearm inward</u> so you keep your palm facing downward as much as possible. Hold the stretch with your elbow extended (Figure 28B–E).

The stretch is performed properly when you feel tension (not pain) in the anterior part of the arm.

Remember to note in your personal log the total number of minutes that you perform this stretching posture each day.

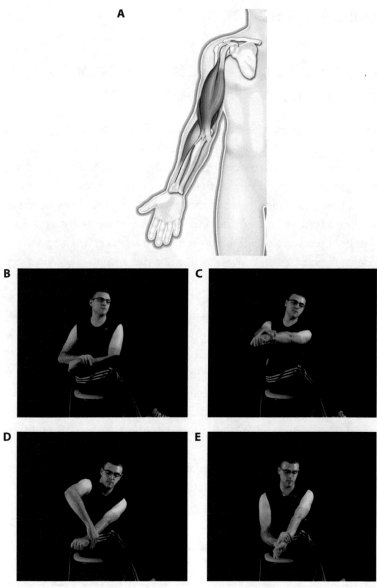

Figure 28

≥ -- minutes ≥ -- times per day

ELBOW – Sheet 29

Elbow flexors – Active elbow extension

Active elbow extension, with the shoulder flexed, is a movement we use to point fingers or grasp an object positioned high in front of us. This movement stretches the elbow flexors (mainly biceps brachii, brachialis anterior, and brachioradialis), which may then oppose elbow extension. The objective is thus to diminish the resistance coming from the elbow flexors to improve amplitude, strength, and speed of elbow extension movements.

The best way to achieve this objective is to repeat sets of active elbow extension exercises (shoulder flexed) of maximum amplitude and speed every day.

This workout is best done while standing in front of a wall – or seated if the standing position is impossible – on which a target has been marked <u>at maximum height</u> reachable. Importantly, the distance between the wall and your feet should be <u>the maximum distance</u> that still allows you to barely reach the target. The movement of the hand starts from the nose, or chest, with the elbow up to the side, reaching for the target and back with each repetition (Figure 29A–C). Ideally, alternate sets of this exercise with elbow flexor stretching postures (Sheet 28), as recommended by your therapist.

Note: For optimal elbow extension movement, the elbow flexors need to be long and well relaxed, which is why your therapist will ask you to stretch them (Sheet 28) and your doctor may suggest injections into these muscles with a neuromuscular blocker.

Please note in your personal log the maximum number of active elbow extensions performed in --- seconds per set.

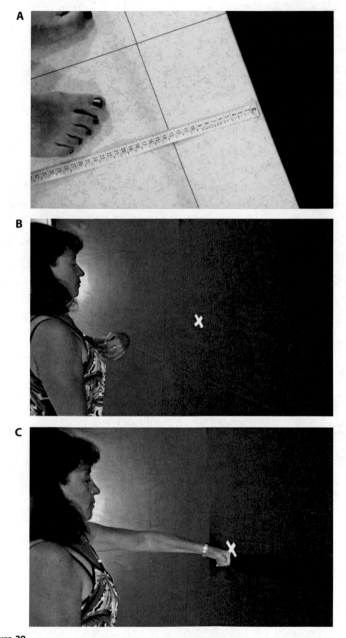

Figure 29

Maximum repetitions in -- seconds, -- times per day

ELBOW – Sheet 30

Pronator quadratus – Passive stretch

The pronator quadratus muscle is located in the forearm close to the wrist (Figure 30A). The pronator quadratus turns the palm downward, whether the elbow is bent or extended. If this muscle is overactive or too short:

- It impedes elbow supination (turning the palm up), which is essential to grasp and use most daily objects, particularly vertical objects placed close to the body (bottle and glass among others) or objects you need to turn to use them (key and spoon among others)
- A short pronator quadratus particularly hinders the supination of the bent elbow (for grasping or using objects close to the body).

The pronator quadratus **stretching posture** can be achieved while sitting with the elbow bent, <u>grasping the wrist – not the hand – from below, and twisting your forearm outward so you keep your palm facing upward as much as possible</u> (Figure 30B–D).

The stretch is performed properly when you feel tension (not pain) in the lower part of the forearm.

Remember to note in your personal log the total number of minutes that you perform this stretching posture each day.

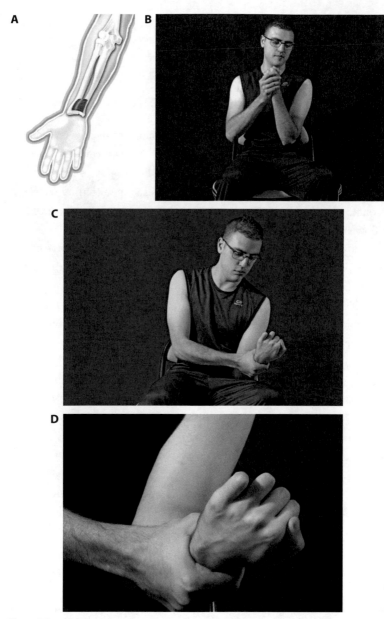

Figure 30

≥ -- minutes ≥ -- times per day

ELBOW – Sheet 31

Pronator quadratus – Active supination, elbow flexed

Supination of the flexed elbow is the movement we use every time we turn a key or grasp a vertical object close by. This movement stretches the pronator quadratus muscle, which may then oppose elbow supination. The objective is thus to diminish the resistance coming from the pronator quadratus to improve the amplitude, strength, and speed of elbow supination with the elbow flexed.

The best way to achieve this objective is to repeat sets of active elbow supination exercises (elbow flexed) of maximum amplitude and speed every day.

This workout is performed while sitting at a table close to the body, the table being low enough – or your chair high enough – for the elbow to rest on it comfortably when flexed. Start with the palm of your hand facing downward. With each repetition <u>try to turn your hand back over</u> (so your palm is facing upward) by attempting to bring your thumb out as much as possible and touching the table if you can. <u>Then turn the palm of your hand downward again</u>, and repeat as many times as possible in each set (Figure 31A–D). Ideally, alternate sets of this exercise with pronator quadratus stretching postures (Sheet 30), as recommended by your therapist.

Note: For optimal elbow supination movements with the elbow flexed, the pronator quadratus needs to be long and well relaxed, which is why your therapist will ask you to stretch it (Sheet 30) and your doctor may suggest injections into this muscle with a neuromuscular blocker.

> **Please note in your log the maximum number of active elbow supinations, elbow flexed performed in --- seconds per set.**

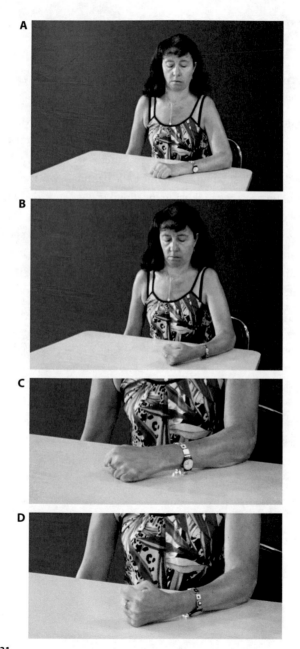

Figure 31

Maximum repetitions in -- seconds, -- times per day

ELBOW – Sheet 32

Pronator teres – Passive stretch

The pronator teres muscle is located in the forearm near the elbow (Figure 32A). The pronator teres turns the palm downward only when the elbow is extended. If this muscle is overactive or too short:

- It impedes elbow supination (turning the palm up), which is essential for grasping and using most daily objects, particularly vertical objects placed far from the body (bottle and glass among others) or objects you need to turn to used them (key and spoon among others)
- A short pronator teres specifically hinders the supination of the straightened elbow (for grasping or using objects far from the body).

The stretching posture is performed in a sitting position while crossing your legs and bending forward at the waist. Place your elbow on the opposite knee. Using your other hand, grab your wrist (Figure 32B) – not your hand – and extend your elbow, <u>twisting your forearm outward</u> so you keep your palm facing upward as much as possible. Hold the stretch with your elbow extended (Figure 32C). Alternatively, the stretching posture can be achieved while sitting at a table and placing the extended elbow on a stack of books in front of you (Figure 32D).

The stretch is performed properly when you feel tension (not pain) in the front part of the arm in the inner elbow.

Remember to note in your personal log the total number of minutes that you perform this stretching posture each day.

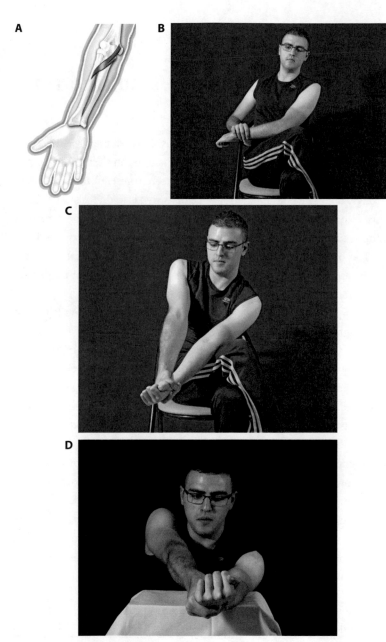

Figure 32

≥ -- minutes ≥ -- times per day

ELBOW – Sheet 33

Pronator teres – Active supination, elbow extended

Active supination with an extended elbow is the movement we use every time we grasp a vertical object placed at a distance on a table (eg, glass or cup). This movement stretches the pronator teres muscle, which may then strongly oppose elbow supination. The objective is to diminish the resistance coming from the pronator teres to improve the amplitude, strength, and speed of elbow supination movements with the elbow extended.

The best way to achieve this objective is to repeat sets of active elbow supination exercises (elbow extended) of maximum amplitude and speed every day.

This particularly difficult workout is performed while sitting at a table high enough for the elbow to rest on it comfortably away from the body. The hand movement starts from the palm positioned on the table (palm facing downward) followed by turning the palm to face upwards. Try to rotate your thumb out as much as possible while keeping your elbow extended. Even if the movement is incomplete, what matters is to go as far out as possible with each movement. You then return the hand back to the palm facing downward position as many times as possible in each set (Figure 33A–D). Ideally, alternate sets of this exercise with pronator teres stretching postures (Sheet 32), as recommended by your therapist.

Note: For optimal elbow supination movements with the elbow extended, both the pronator quadratus and pronator teres need to be long and well relaxed, which is why your therapist will ask you to stretch them (Sheets 30 and 32) and your doctor may suggest injections into these muscles with a neuromuscular blocker.

Please note in your log the maximum number of active elbow supinations elbow extended performed in --- seconds per set.

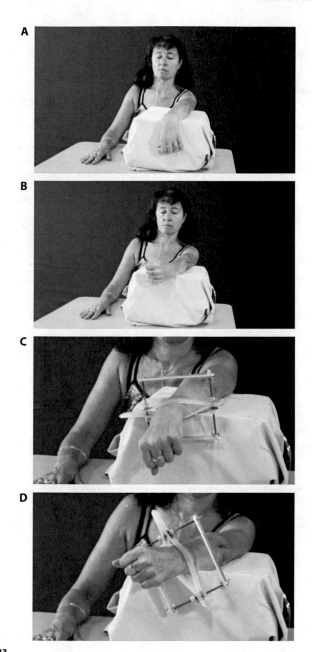

Figure 33

Maximum repetitions in -- seconds, -- times per day

WRIST – Sheet 34

Wrist flexors – Passive stretch

The wrist flexor muscles are located in the front part of the forearm. The two main wrist flexors are flexor carpi radialis on the outside and flexor carpi ulnaris on the inside. Many other muscles help to flex the wrist including the palmaris longus (which also cups the hand) and all the forearm-located finger flexors (flexor digitorum superficialis and profundus and flexor pollicis longus Figure 34A). Flexor carpi radialis only flexes the wrist, while flexor carpi ulnaris flexes the wrist and deviates it inwards.

If these muscles are overactive or too short, they impede wrist extension. Wrist extension is essential for any grasping activity because bending your fingers to grasp an object is always performed with the wrist slightly extended.

To perform this stretching posture, sit with your elbow flexed, ideally with both elbows (at least the paretic elbow) laid on a table or on your hips. Grab the hand, placing it palm to palm with your other hand and pull your paretic hand upward, trying to extend your wrist backwards as much as possible (Figure 34B–D).

This stretch is performed properly when you feel tension (not pain) in the front part of the forearm.

Remember to note in your personal log the total number of minutes that you perform this stretching posture each day.

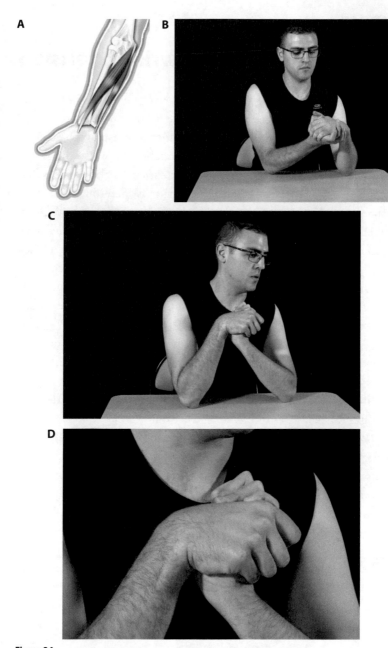

Figure 34

≥ -- minutes ≥ -- times per day

WRIST – Sheet 35

Wrist flexors – Active wrist extension

The movement of active wrist extension is one you use every time you catch and grasp an object. Indeed, wrist extension must be coordinated with the action of the finger flexors in order to grasp an object with maximum efficiency. This movement stretches the wrist and finger flexor muscles, which then oppose wrist extension. The objective is thus to diminish the resistance coming from the wrist and finger flexors to improve the amplitude, strength, and speed of wrist extension movements.

The best way to achieve this objective is to repeat sets of active wrist extension exercises (fingers flexed, and then fingers extended when possible) of maximum amplitude and speed every day.

This workout is performed while sitting. The hand movement starts with the wrist flexed over the edge of a table, first with the hand open if possible, trying to <u>lift your hand with straight fingers off the plane of the table</u> (Figure 35A). If this is impossible, try lifting up the hand with the fingers flexed at each movement (Figure 35B). Then the hand returns back down and so on, as many times as possible in each set. Ideally, alternate sets of this exercise with the wrist flexors stretching postures (Sheet 34), as recommended by your therapist.

Note: For optimal wrist extension movements, the flexor carpi radialis, flexor carpi ulnaris, palmaris longus, flexor digitorum profundus/superficialis, and flexor pollicis longus need to be long and well relaxed, which is why your therapist will ask you to stretch them (Sheets 34, 36, 37, and 42) and your doctor may suggest injections into these muscles with a neuromuscular blocker.

Please note in your log the maximum number of active wrist extensions, fingers extended or fingers flexed, performed in --- seconds per set.

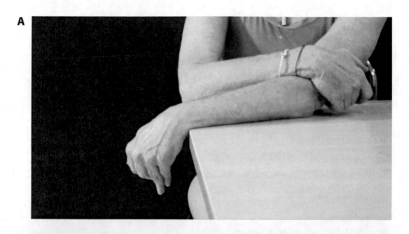

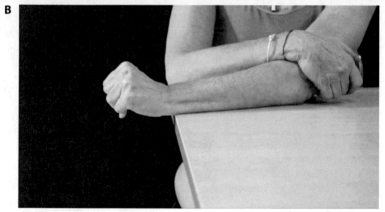

Figure 35

Maximum repetitions in -- seconds, -- times per day

HAND – Sheet 36

Flexors of digits II and III – Passive stretch

Flexor digitorum superficialis and profundus of digits II and III are located in the front part of the forearm (Figure 36A). These muscles flex the second and third fingers, and also help to flex the wrist.

If these muscles are overactive or too short, they impede second and third finger extension, which is an essential prerequisite to grasping, particularly for larger objects.

The stretching posture can be achieved while sitting, holding the second and third fingers with your other hand, and trying to pull the fingers backward. Try to keep your wrist extended as much as possible (Figure 36B–D).

This stretch is performed properly when you feel tension (not pain) in the front part of the forearm.

> **Remember to note in your personal log the total number of minutes that you perform this stretching posture each day.**

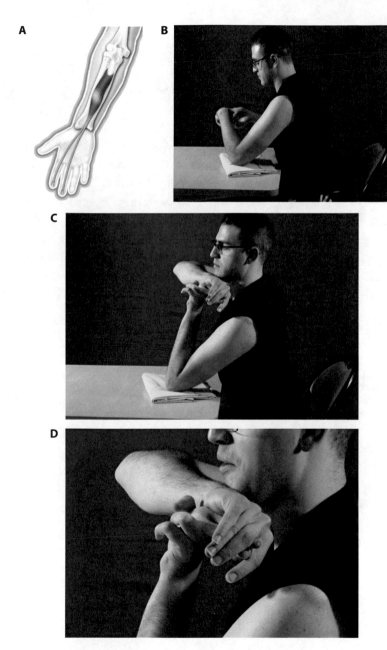

Figure 36

≥ -- minutes ≥ -- times per day

HAND – Sheet 37

Flexors of digits IV and V – Passive stretch

Flexor digitorum superficialis and profundus of digits IV and V are located in the front part of the forearm (Figure 37A). These muscles flex the fourth and fifth fingers and also help to flex the wrist.

If these muscles are overactive or too short, they impede fourth and fifth finger extension, which is an essential prerequisite to grasping, particularly for long and narrow objects (fork and broom among others).

The stretching posture can be achieved while sitting, holding the fourth and fifth fingers with your other hand, and trying to pull the fingers backward. Keep your wrist extended as much as possible during the stretch (Figure 37B–D).

This stretch is performed properly when you feel tension (not pain) in the front part of the forearm.

Remember to note in your personal log the total number of minutes that you perform this stretching posture each day.

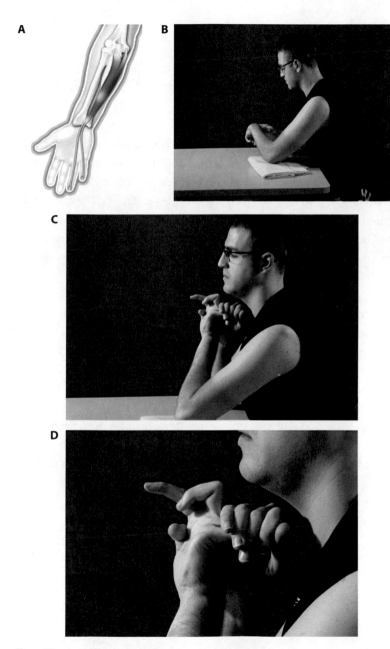

Figure 37

≥ -- minutes ≥ -- times per day

HAND – Sheet 38

Flexors of digits II–V – Active whole hand opening

Active extension of all fingers is used to catch or manipulate large objects (for example a ball, cup, bottle, or shoe). This movement stretches the flexor digitorum profundus, flexor digitorum superficialis, and interosseus muscles of all fingers, which then oppose finger extension. The objective is thus to diminish the resistance coming from the flexor digitorum profundus, flexor digitorum superficialis, lumbricals, and interosseus muscles to improve the amplitude, strength, and speed of hand opening movements.

The best way to achieve this objective is to repeat sets of active hand opening exercises of maximum amplitude and speed every day.

This workout is performed while sitting. Start from a position with the wrist kept fully flexed by your other hand (Figure 38A–B). When this exercise gets easier, start with your wrist straight (neutral), fist clenched, and try to <u>open your hand as wide as possible</u> (Figure 38C–D). Ideally, alternate sets of this exercise with finger flexors stretching postures (Sheets 36, 37, and 40), as recommended by your therapist.

Note: For optimal hand opening movements, the flexor digitorum profundus, flexor digitorum superficialis, and interosseus muscles need to be long and thoroughly relaxed, which is why your therapist will ask you to stretch them (Sheets 36, 37, and 40) and your doctor may suggest injections into these muscles with a neuromuscular blocker.

Please note in your personal log the maximum number of hand opening movements performed in --- seconds per set.

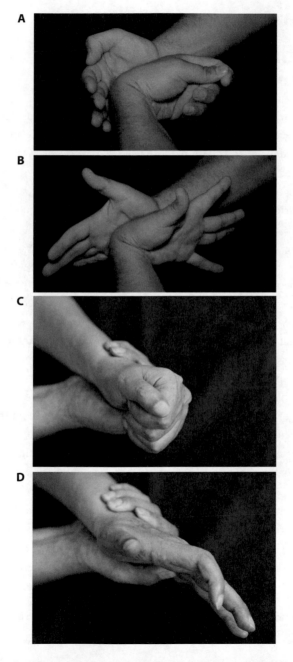

Figure 38

HAND – Sheet 39

Flexors of digits II–V – Active extension of each digit

Active extension of an individual finger is used to catch or manipulate small objects (for example, fork, spoon, coin, button, shoelace, or pen) and is also used together with the extension of the other fingers when grasping large objects (cup or bottle among others). This movement stretches the flexor digitorum profundus, flexor digitorum superficialis, and interosseus muscles, which then oppose finger extension. The objective is thus to diminish the resistance coming from the flexor digitorum profundus, flexor digitorum superficialis, and interosseus muscles to improve the amplitude, strength and speed of individual finger opening movements.

The best way to achieve this objective is to repeat sets of active individual finger extension exercises of maximum amplitude and speed every day.

This workout is performed while sitting. Start from a position where your wrist and fingers are flexed over the edge of the table (Figure 39A–B) or around an object and raise each finger (one finger at a time) as high as possible. When this exercise gets easier, place your palm down on the table with fingers extended (Figure 39C–D). Raise each finger (one finger at a time) as high off the table as possible without the other fingers leaving the table (Figure 39A–D shows an example for the index finger). If necessary use the other hand to keep the other fingers on the table). Ideally, alternate sets of this exercise with finger flexor stretching postures (Sheets 36, 37, and 40), as recommended by your therapist.

Note: For optimal active finger extension movements, the flexor digitorum profundus, flexor digitorum superficialis, and interosseus muscles need to be long and thoroughly relaxed, which is why your therapist will ask you to stretch them (Sheets 36 and 37) and your doctor may suggest injections into these muscles with a neuromuscular blocker.

Please note in your log the maximum number of active finger extensions performed in --- seconds per set.

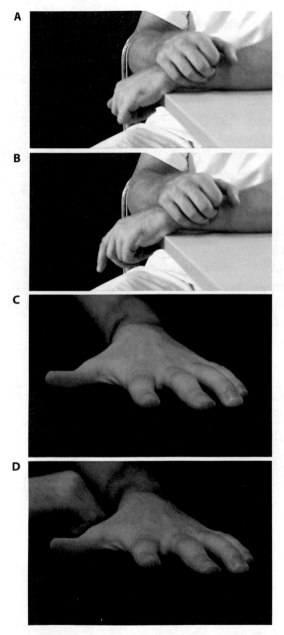

Figure 39

Maximum repetitions in -- seconds, -- times per day

HAND – Sheet 40

Interosseus muscles – Passive stretch

Palmar and dorsal interosseous muscles are located inside the hand between the metacarpal bones, which join the wrist to the first phalanx of the fingers. These muscles flex the first joint of the fingers (metacarpophalangeal joint, Figure 40A).

If these muscles are overactive or too short, they impede finger extension, which is an essential prerequisite to grasping, particularly for larger objects.

The stretching posture can be achieved while sitting, firmly holding the first phalanx of the second to fifth fingers with the whole of the other hand, and trying to pull the first phalanx backward, tips of fingers may bend (Figure 40B–D). <u>The wrist should remain flexed</u> and not involved in the stretch.

The stretch is performed properly when you feel tension (not pain) in the higher part of the palm.

Remember to note in your personal log the total number of minutes that you perform this stretching posture each day.

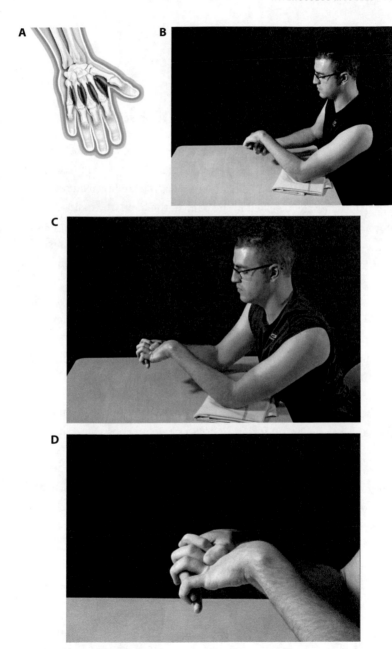

Figure 40

≥ -- minutes ≥ -- times per day

HAND – Sheet 41

Interosseus muscles – Active extension of the first phalanx

When you are about to grasp a large object, you must be able to open the hand sufficiently. This action is performed thanks to a muscle group called extensor digitorum communis as well as the lumbrical muscles. The interosseus muscles (located in the palm of the hand, the main intrinsic muscles) can oppose this action as they tend to flex the first phalanx of the fingers towards the palm. The objective is thus to diminish the resistance coming from the interosseus muscles to improve amplitude, strength, and speed of hand opening movements.

The best way to achieve this objective is to repeat sets of active first phalanx extension exercises of the fingers II to V, of maximum amplitude and speed every day.

This workout is performed while sitting, <u>with the wrist blocked into full flexion</u> using the other hand. You must try to extend the first phalanx of the fingers as much as possible with each repetition, keeping the other phalangeal joints bent (Figure 41A–C). Ideally, alternate sets of this exercise with interosseus muscles stretching postures (Sheet 40), as recommended by your therapist.

Note: For optimal active first phalanx extension movements, the interosseus muscles need to be long and well relaxed, which is why your therapist will ask you to stretch them (Sheet 40) and your doctor may suggest injections into these muscles with a neuromuscular blocker.

Please note in your log the maximum number of active first phalanx extensions performed in --- seconds per set.

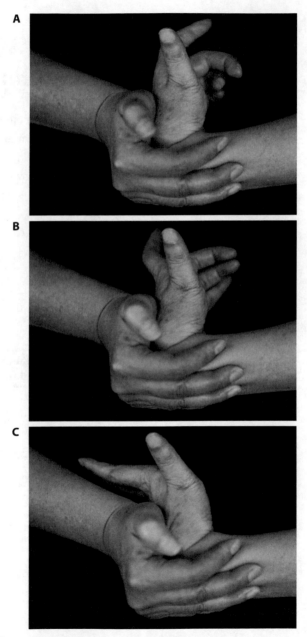

Figure 41

Maximum repetitions in -- seconds, -- times per day

THUMB – Sheet 42

Long thumb flexor – Passive stretch

The long thumb flexor (flexor pollicis longus) is located in the outer part of the forearm (Figure 42A). It bends the distal phalanx of thumb and contributes to the movement of the thumb inward to the palm.

If this muscle is hyperactive or too short, it hinders the movement of the thumb away from the palm (abduction/extension), which is required to enable grasping (especially of large objects).

The stretching posture can be achieved while sitting. Grab your thumb with your other hand (use your whole hand) and pull it upward and backward. Try to keep your wrist extended during this stretch if you can (Figure 42B).

This stretch is performed properly when you feel tension (not pain) in the thumb and the forearm.

Remember to note in your personal log the total number of minutes that you perform this stretching posture each day.

A

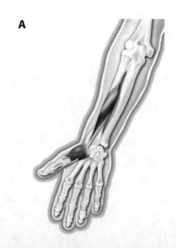

B

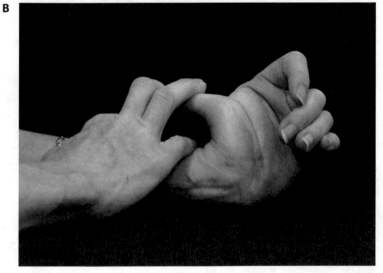

Figure 42

≥ -- minutes ≥ -- times per day

THUMB – Sheet 43

Long thumb flexor – Active long thumb extension

The active thumb extension movement is indispensable when using your hand to catch and manipulate small (for example, button, spoon, shoelace, or pen) or large objects (for example, cup or bottle). This movement stretches the flexor pollicis longus muscle, which may then oppose thumb extension. The objective is thus to diminish the resistance coming from the long thumb flexor muscle (flexor pollicis longus) to improve amplitude, strength, and speed of individual thumb opening movements.

The best way to achieve this objective is to repeat sets of active thumb extension/abductions exercises of maximum amplitude and speed every day.

This workout is performed while sitting. The movement may start with your wrist and fingers bent over the edge of the table or around an object. Try to <u>lift up and spread the thumb apart from the hand</u> as many times as possible without lifting up the hand or the other fingers. When this exercise gets easier, hold your wrist in a neutral position with your other hand and try to lift up the thumb as much as possible (Figure 43). Ideally, alternate sets of this exercise with long thumb flexor stretching postures (Sheet 42), as recommended by your therapist.

Note: For optimal active long thumb extension movements, the flexor pollicis longus needs to be long and well relaxed, which is why your therapist will ask you to stretch it (Sheet 42) and your doctor may suggest injections into these muscles with a neuromuscular blocker.

> **Please note in your personal log the maximum number of active long thumb extensions, performed in --- seconds per set.**

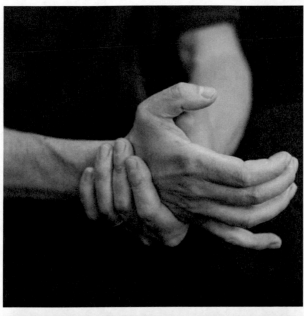

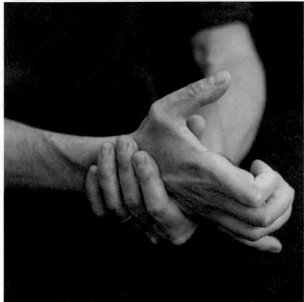

Figure 43

Maximum repetitions in -- seconds, -- times per day

THUMB – Sheet 44

Short thumb flexor – Passive stretch

The short thumb flexor (flexor pollicis brevis) is located deep in the outer part of the palm (thenar eminence; Figure 44A). It contributes to the bending of the thumb inward into the palm.

If this muscle is hyperactive or too short, it hinders the movement of the thumb away from the palm (extension), which is required to enable grasping (especially of large objects).

The stretching posture can be achieved while sitting. With your other hand (use your whole hand) <u>block the wrist into full flexion</u>, grab, and push the first phalanx of your thumb upward and backward. Try to keep your wrist bent during this stretch (Figure 44B).

This stretch is performed properly when you feel tension (not pain) in the thumb and the palm.

Remember to note in your personal log the total number of minutes that you perform this stretching posture each day.

A

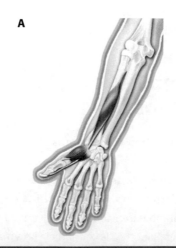

B

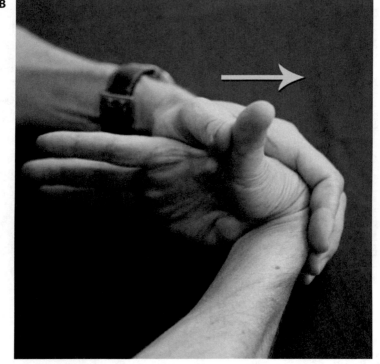

Figure 44

≥ -- minutes ≥ -- times per day

THUMB – Sheet 45

Short thumb flexor – Active short thumb extension

The active thumb extension movement is indispensable when using your hand to catch and manipulate small (for example, button, spoon, shoelace, or pen) or large objects (for example, cup or bottle). The movement practiced here stretches the flexor pollicis brevis muscle, which may then oppose thumb extension. The objective is thus to diminish the resistance coming from the flexor pollicis brevis muscle to improve amplitude, strength, and speed of individual thumb opening movements.

The best way to achieve this objective is to repeat sets of active thumb extension exercises of maximum amplitude and speed every day.

This workout is performed while sitting and <u>keeping your wrist fully bent with your other hand</u>. Try to lift up the thumb as many times as possible (Figure 45). Ideally, alternate sets of this exercise with flexor pollicis brevis stretching postures (Sheet 44), as recommended by your therapist.

Note: For optimal active short thumb extension movements, the flexor pollicis brevis needs to be long and well relaxed, which is why your therapist will ask you to stretch it (Sheet 44) and your doctor may suggest injections into these muscles with a neuromuscular blocker.

Please note in your personal log the maximum number of active short thumb extensions, performed in --- seconds per set.

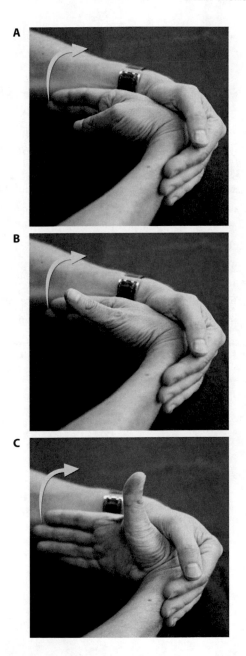

Figure 45

Maximum repetitions in -- seconds, -- times per day

THUMB – Sheet 46

Opponens pollicis – Passive stretch

The thumb opponent (opponens pollicis) is located in the central and outer part of the palm (thenar eminence; (Figure 46A). It moves the thumb inward to the palm.

If this muscle is hyperactive or too short, it hinders the movement of the thumb away from the palm (de-opposition), which is required to enable grasping (especially of large objects) or to release objects.

The stretching posture can be achieved while sitting. Pull the <u>proximal</u> part of your thumb as much as possible outward with the other hand (Figure 46B–C).

This stretch is performed properly when you feel tension (not pain) in the thumb and the central and outer part of the palm.

Remember to note in your personal log the total number of minutes that you perform this stretching posture each day.

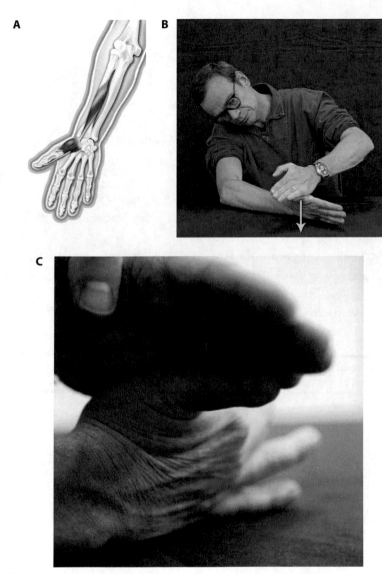

Figure 46

≥ -- minutes ≥ -- times per day

THUMB – Sheet 47

Long abductor of the thumb – Passive stretch

The long abductor of the thumb (abductor pollicis longus) is located in the back part of the forearm (Figure 47A). It moves the thumb outward away from the palm.

If this muscle is hyperactive or too short, it hinders the movement of the thumb towards the palm (opposition), which is required to enable grasping (especially of small objects).

The stretching posture can be achieved while sitting. Pull the proximal part of your thumb towards the palm, <u>while blocking your wrist into full flexion</u> (Figure 47B–C).

This stretch is performed properly when you feel tension (not pain) in the thumb and the back part of the forearm.

> **Remember to note in your personal log the total number of minutes that you perform this stretching posture each day.**

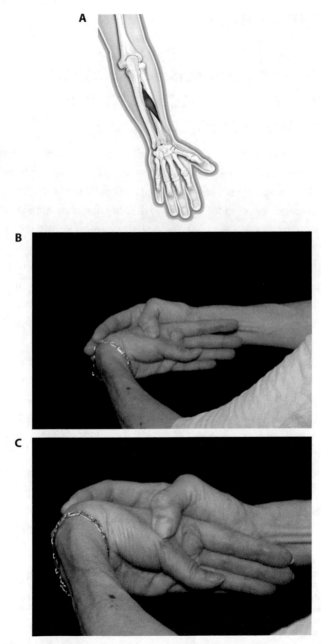

Figure 47

≥ -- minutes ≥ -- times per day

THUMB – Sheet 48

Opponens pollicis/Long abductor of the thumb – Active thumb deopposition/opposition

The active thumb deopposition movement is indispensable when using your hand to catch and manipulate large objects (for example, cup or bottle). The movement stretches the opponens pollicis muscle (the opposite movement – opposition – stretches the long abductor of the thumb). The objective is thus to diminish the resistance coming from the opponens pollicis muscle (or from the long abductor) to improve amplitude, strength, and speed of individual thumb opening (or closing) movements.

The best way to achieve this objective is to repeat sets of active thumb deopposition/opposition exercises of maximum amplitude and speed every day.

This workout is performed while sitting. *For deopposition exercises*, <u>try to spread the thumb apart from the hand in an arching movement</u> as many times as possible; *for opposition exercises*, try to bring the thumb inward towards the plan in an arching movement as many times as possible (Figure 48A–C). Ideally, alternate sets of this exercise with the opponens pollicis stretching postures (Sheet 46) – or with the long abductor stretching postures (Sheet 47) – as recommended by your therapist.

Note: For optimal active thumb deopposition/opposition movements, the oponens pollicis/long abductor of the thumb needs to be long and well relaxed, which is why your therapist will ask you to stretch it (Sheet 46 or Sheet 47) and your doctor may suggest injections into these muscles with a neuromuscular blocker.

Please note in your personal log the maximum number of active thumb deoppositions/oppositions performed in --- seconds per set.

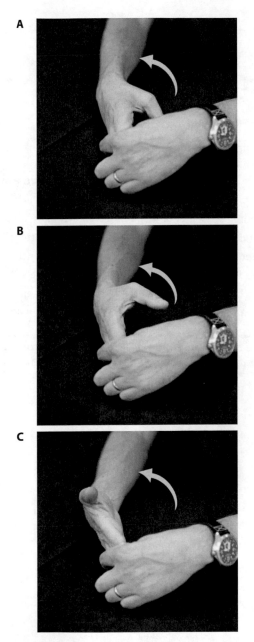

Figure 48

Maximum repetitions in -- seconds, -- times per day

THUMB – Sheet 49

Adductor pollicis – Passive stretch

The thumb adductor (adductor pollicis) is located in the outer part of the palm (thenar eminence; Figure 49A). It moves the thumb inward toward the second finger.

If this muscle is hyperactive or too short, it hinders the movement of the thumb away from the other fingers (abduction), which is required to enable grasping (especially of large objects) or release objects.

The stretching posture can be achieved while sitting. Pull the first metacarp (not the first phalanx of the thumb) away from the second finger using a firm grip with thumb and index (Figure 49B).

This stretch is performed properly when you feel tension (not pain) in the thumb and the space between the thumb and the index finger.

Remember to note in your personal log the total number of minutes that you perform this stretching posture each day.

A

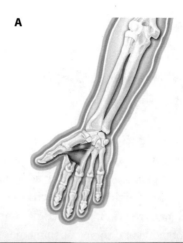

B

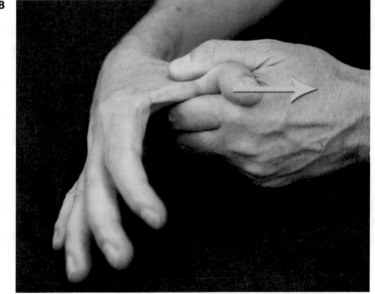

Figure 49

≥ -- minutes ≥ -- times per day

THUMB – Sheet 50

Adductor pollicis – Active short thumb abduction

The active thumb short abduction movement is indispensable when using your hand to catch and manipulate large objects (for example, cup or bottle). This movement stretches the thumb adductor muscle, which may then oppose thumb abduction. The objective is thus to diminish the resistance coming from the thumb adductor to improve amplitude, strength, and speed of individual thumb opening movements.

The best way to achieve this objective is to repeat sets of active thumb short abduction exercises of maximum amplitude and speed every day.

This workout is performed while sitting. Try to spread the thumb horizontally from the palm as many times as possible (Figure 50A–C). Ideally, alternate sets of this exercise with the thumb adductor stretching postures (Sheet 49), as recommended by your therapist.

Note: For optimal active thumb extension movements, the adductor pollicis needs to be long and well relaxed, which is why your therapist will ask you to stretch it (Sheet 49) and your doctor may suggest injections into this muscle with a neuromuscular blocker.

Please note in your personal log the maximum number of active short thumb abductions, performed in --- seconds per set.

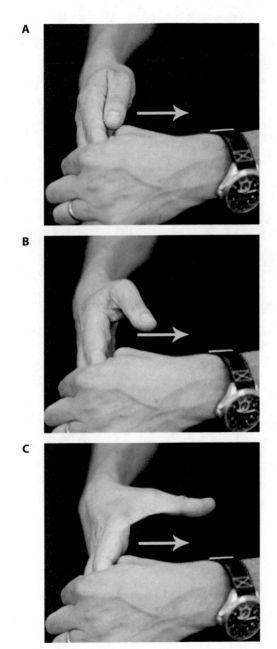

Figure 50

Maximum repetitions in -- seconds, -- times per day

Appendix

Personal log sheet – Lower limb

HIP	N°											
Dates												
Gluteus maximus:												
Passive stretch (min)												
Hip flexion, knee flexed (nb of mvts)												
Hamstrings:												
Passive stretch (min)												
Hip flexion, knee extended (nb of mvts)												
Hip flexor-adductors:												
Passive stretch (min)												
Hip extensor-adductors:												
Passive stretch (min)												
Hip abduction (nb of mvts)												
Hip internal rotators:												
Passive stretch (min)												
Hip external rotation (nb of mvts)												

Personal log sheet – Lower limb

KNEE							
Nº Dates							
Rectus femoris:							
Passive stretch (min)							
Knee flexion, hip extended (nb of mvts)							
Vastus muscles:							
Passive stretch (min)							
Knee flexion, hip flexed (nb of mvts)							

ANKLE							
Nº Dates							
Soleus:							
Passive stretch (min)							
Ankle dorsiflexion, seated (nb of mvts)							
Gastrocnemius (medial and lateral):							
Passive stretch (min)							
Ankle dorsiflexion, standing (nb of mvts)							

Personal log sheet – Lower limb

LOWER LIMB FUNCTIONAL EXERCISES													
N° Dates													
Sit-to-stand													
Long stride walking													
Fast walking													

Personal log sheet – Upper limb

SHOULDER											
N° Dates											
Pectoralis major:											
Passive stretch (min)											
Shoulder abduction (nb of mvts)											
Latissimus dorsi and long head of triceps:											
Passive stretch (min)											
Latissimus dorsi:											
Shoulder flexion, elbow extended (nb of mvts)											
Long head of triceps:											
Shoulder flexion, elbow flexed (nb of mvts)											
Sub-scapularis:											
Passive stretch (min)											
Shoulder external rotation (nb of mvts)											

Personal log sheet – Upper limb

ELBOW												
N°	**Dates**											
Elbow flexors:												
Passive stretch (min)												
Elbow extension (nb of mvts)												
Pronator quadratus:												
Passive stretch (min)												
Supination, elbow flexed (nb of mvts)												
Pronator teres:												
Passive stretch (min)												
Supination, elbow extended (nb of mvts)												

WRIST					
N°	**Dates**				
Wrist flexors:					
Passive stretch (min)					
Wrist extension (nb of mvts)					

Personal log sheet – Upper limb

HAND										
N°	Dates									
Flexors of digits II and III:										
Passive stretch (min)										
Flexors of digits IV and V:										
Passive stretch (min)										
Flexors of digits II–V:										
Whole hand opening (nb of mvts)										
Extension of each digit (nb of mvts)										
Interosseus muscles:										
Passive stretch (min)										
Extension of the first phalanx (nb of mvts)										

Personal log sheet – Upper limb

THUMB																	
N° **Dates**																	
Long thumb flexor:																	
Passive stretch (min)																	
Long thumb extension (nb of mvts)																	
Short thumb flexor:																	
Passive stretch (min)																	
Short thumb extension (nb of mvts)																	
Opponens pollicis:																	
Passive stretch (min)																	
Long abductor of the thumb:																	
Passive stretch (min)																	
Opponens pollicis/Long abductor of the thumb:																	
Thumb deopposition/opposition (nb of mvts)																	
Adductor pollicis:																	
Passive stretch (min)																	
Short thumb abduction (nb of mvts)																	

Neuroloco

Reconquering Movement

www.neuroloco.org

(Non-profit association)

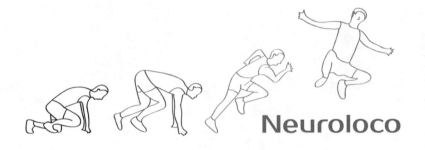

Promoting Research in Neurorehabilitation and Orthopedic Rehabilitation

Contact:
Hôpitaux Universitaires Henri Mondor
Service de Rééducation Neurolocomotrice
40 rue de Mesly, 94000 Créteil, France
Tél : +33-1-49-81-30-61
www.neuroloco.org

Printed in the United States
by Baker & Taylor Publisher Services